# THE OZEMPIC REVOLUTION

# THE OZEMPIC REVOLUTION

A Doctor's Proven Plan for Success
to Help You Reverse Obesity,
End Yo-Yo Dieting, and Protect
Yourself from Disease

## ALEXANDRA SOWA, MD

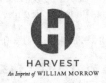

HARVEST
*An Imprint of* WILLIAM MORROW

THE OZEMPIC REVOLUTION. Copyright © 2025 by Alexandra Sowa. All rights reserved. Printed in the United States of America. No part of this book may be used or reproduced in any manner whatsoever without written permission except in the case of brief quotations embodied in critical articles and reviews. For information, address HarperCollins Publishers, 195 Broadway, New York, NY 10007.

HarperCollins books may be purchased for educational, business, or sales promotional use. For information, please email the Special Markets Department at SPsales@harpercollins.com.

FIRST EDITION

Library of Congress Cataloging-in-Publication Data has been applied for.

ISBN 978-0-06-341700-7

24 25 26 27 28 LBC 5 4 3 2 1

To Peter and our four *why*s:
Peter George, Henry, Brooks, and Adele

# Contents

## SECTION III
# Your GLP-1 Life

## SECTION IV
# Recipes and Dining Out

# In Conclusion
### 199

# Why Doctors Have Failed You

When I decided to enter training to become an obesity medicine specialist, I got grimaces from some colleagues. There were comments along the lines of, "Wow, *why*? I hate dealing with those people." By *those people*, they meant people with obesity, who carry significant excess weight—which is about 43 percent of the US population.

I guess I shouldn't have been surprised that doctors, like many—or even most—people in our society, would be guilty of weight stigma. Still, it upset me. Doctors have tremendous power over their patients' well-being, and every doctor takes a pledge to do no harm. If you've been on the receiving end of weight stigma, you know that it causes great harm.

My patients tell me stories that shock me. They might go to the doctor complaining of acute pain, but instead of listening, the physician rudely interrupts them to talk about their weight. Instead of feeling seen and supported, the patient feels ignored. Instead of being cared for, they are shamed. So—no surprise—many just stop going to the doctor.

Doctors absolutely *love* to recommend weight loss, but the irony is that they're often not very qualified to give advice on it. Historically, medical students and residents have received hardly any training on nutrition. Most doctors gave the same advice to their patients that I got as a young adult whose weight hovered near the top of the healthy range: "Move more, eat less." They might have given you a quick talk or a handout on nutrition, which amounted to a regurgitation of the USDA's guidelines. The advice tended to be tone-deaf and lacking in substance. And yet when their patients failed to lose weight and keep it off, who did the doctors blame? You guessed it: the patients.

Until very recently, doctors have regarded excess weight primarily as a failure of willpower. Overweight people have often been seen as victims of their own sloth, ignorance, or some combination of the two. Thanks to research in my field, we now know that obesity is a fact of biology. It's a disease state, and I'll explain in chapter 1 why it so often requires medical intervention to reverse.

But we also know obesity is complicated. Weight gain is multi-factorial, meaning it's not usually caused by just one thing. This also makes it legitimately hard for doctors to provide effective treatment. The 20-minute visits that are standard in our healthcare system don't provide enough time for doctors and their patients to unravel the mix of issues, both physical and psychological, that can complicate maintaining a healthy weight.

As a doctor who works exclusively with individuals who carry significant excess weight, I know we can't ignore those mental and physical issues and be successful. But I also know this: All this complexity, all this stigma, is exactly why glucagon-like peptide-1 (GLP-1) agonist drugs—such as Ozempic, Wegovy, Mounjaro, and Zepbound—are the most powerful, life-changing, lifesaving tool I have to offer my patients.

The patients I see in my practice have all kinds of histories that have contributed to their excess weight—and yet the GLP-1 drugs work for pretty much *all of them*. That includes people like Alice, who was recovering from a binge-eating disorder. Or David, a lifetime marathoner who had been sidelined by spinal stenosis and needed to return to a healthy weight for corrective surgery. Or Catherine, who couldn't lose weight after pregnancy. I help women who need to lose weight so they can start fertility treatment. Patients dealing with weight gain from cancer protocols. Patients recovering from sexual trauma. Lifetime chronic dieters. Recovering alcoholics who replaced booze with food. And still more people who can't pinpoint why, but who know the number on the scale went up over 50 pounds in the past ten years and now *will . . . not . . . budge.*

Universally, my patients on GLP-1s feel incredible relief when the drugs prove to them that a correctable health condition has kept them from losing weight. Their food noise—the voice in their head that is relentlessly focused on what they should eat next—shuts off, to their great relief. After many years or a lifetime of constantly restricting themselves, they finally get to feel what it's like to put their fork down because they are *satisfied*. When they no longer have to fight biology or fear the scale, they finally feel empowered to deal with other factors that may have contributed to their excess weight. With the help of GLP-1 drugs, we're able to separate the medical from the emotional and behavioral in a profound new way.

## The Promise of GLP-1s

GLP-1 drugs have been remarkably helpful for my patients, and so many others—but you'd never know that from the media coverage. The big story has been all about body image–obsessed celebrities. Or it's been fearmongering headlines about "Ozempic face" or "paralyzed stomach" (the latter being a medically inaccurate description of gastroparesis, an extremely rare adverse event). Because obesity is stigmatized and misunderstood, so are the medicines to treat it.

Naturally, people are nervous and skeptical when they hear about a new "wonder drug," particularly one that has anything to do with weight loss. The last major Food and Drug Administration (FDA)-approved drugs for weight loss were catastrophic fails. In the 1990s, there was fen-phen (fenfluramine/phentermine), a stimulant drug combination that had to be pulled off the shelves when a study confirmed that one of its components, fenfluramine, caused heart valve damage. Later came orlistat, which became better known for producing bowel incontinence than for weight loss. (Poopy pants aside, it wasn't very effective.) But unlike fen-phen and orlistat, GLP-1s have been prescribed by doctors for blood sugar management since 2005 and for weight loss for over a decade, establishing a strong track record for both safety and efficacy. The fen-phen disaster also led to much tougher protocols for the study of drugs before they are released to the public.

Alongside the many medical fails sits the unregulated weight loss industry, which in the US alone is worth more than $20 billion annually[1]—not because it works, but because it doesn't! Commercial weight loss programs have helped some customers lose weight, but the vast majority of dieters have eventually gained back what they've lost, and often added more pounds on top of that (I'll explain this phenomenon in chapter 1).

In this bleak reality, the body positivity movement emerged as an important alternative to diet culture. The concept of "Health at Any Size" has exposed weight stigma in medicine, giving people tools to advocate for themselves and forcing doctors to face their own bias. Hopefully, people of all sizes and ages have less shame around what they look like. Still, beneath these welcome improvements in attitudes is some unchanged science. Overwhelmingly, the evidence links obesity to serious health issues down the road. I'll dig into this topic in chapter 4, but the short story is that a body mass index (BMI) over 30 combined with a large midsection indicates an increased future risk for a variety of illnesses. But as I see it, body positivity and GLP-1 drugs are partners in treating obesity, not adversaries.

Millions of people's health and well-being could benefit significantly from GLP-1 drugs—if they aren't scared away by medical weight stigma, by the skewed information that dominates headlines, by the failures of older weight loss methods, or by the story they heard about their friend's friend's friend who took Wegovy and was so nauseated, they vomited for three days straight. Because here's what the evidence and the collective experience of my patients tells me: *The Ozempic revolution changes everything.* These drugs finally provide a viable, healthy, and reasonable alternative to all of the above. Their use shouldn't be seen as destructive to body positivity, but supportive of it. They aren't another concession to diet culture, but a means to free ourselves from it.

This book combines all the available data with the real-life experiences of patients at my obesity medicine practice, SoWell Health, to help you make an *informed* decision with your doctor about whether you should pursue medical weight management.

## Beyond the Prescription

There's yet another hurdle to reaching the full potential of GLP-1s. These medications are effective—unbelievably effective—but success requires so much more than a prescription. The data illuminates this: Currently, up to 66 percent of people stop taking GLP-1s in less than a year.[2] This means they don't experience the intended benefit, which is long-term, sustainable weight loss that protects them from disease. We need studies to understand why so many people quit taking GLP-1s before reaping the rewards, but as someone who has had great success treating patients with these meds long-term, I see four major reasons.

First, they have unrealistic expectations: Lacking information, they think the weight will fall off right away. In this book, I offer clear data and vivid descriptions of what every point on the GLP-1 journey looks like, setting users up to stay the course for the long haul.

Second, they need help managing side effects: GLP-1 users need to learn how to eat to prevent the most common side effects (nausea, diarrhea, constipation, and fatigue), particularly in the early months when these uncomfortable side effects are most likely. This book provides a new framework for food choices that manages these issues while supporting optimal health.

Third, they lack social support: So many of my patients get nothing but grief from their family and friends (and even their doctors!) about their decision to use GLP-1s. They need information and the self-belief to feel confident and empowered while taking these drugs—none of which comes with their prescription.

And finally, they can't afford it: In the United States, these drugs have had a list price of upward of $1,000 a month. (Compare that to $100 to $200 a month in the United Kingdom and Europe.) Many insurance companies—including Medicaid and Medicare, in most cases—don't cover weight loss drugs, and some that do claim that the costs will soon force them to limit access and length of coverage. This is a definite challenge, but change is coming. Downward pressure on prices is likely as new GLP-1 drugs reach the market. As well, studies demonstrating the long-term benefits for cardiovascular and metabolic health will change the "affordable" equation dramatically. A 2023 study of more than 17,000 people—yes, sponsored by Ozempic manufacturer Novo Nordisk but double-blinded and carried out by top cardiology researchers—has already shown that taking the GLP-1 semaglutide (marketed as Wegovy) cuts the risk of cardiac complications, such as heart attacks and strokes, by 20 percent.[3] As a result, Medicare users with obesity and an existing cardiovascular condition are now eligible for coverage—offering hope that as wider benefits are proven, insurance coverage will continue to expand.

## Introducing the SoWell Method

For GLP-1 users, this book will close that yawning gap between prescription and success. At its center is the SoWell Method, a holistic approach to treating obesity and chronic overweight in combination with

GLP-1s that consolidates 10 years of experience prescribing these medications. You'll find it shares ground with other methods you may have encountered, but it has been completely refocused through the lens of my experience working with thousands of SoWell patients, many of them for multiple years of treatment and maintenance.

The SoWell Method, which can be used to support GLP-1 usage or independently, has three foundations:

1. **Habit Foundations.** These include daily food and mood tracking. My patients recognize many of these habits from previous weight loss attempts, and yet experience them completely differently while on GLP-1s. What they find is that the drugs help them move toward *emotional neutrality* when it comes to their weight, which eases their resistance to embracing new, health-supporting behaviors.

2. **Food Foundations.** Many of my patients experience food satisfaction for the first time in their lives while on GLP-1s. This gives them the space to break free from diet culture oriented on restriction. Instead, they learn to dial up food choices that reduce GLP-1 side effects and increase satisfaction. Where diets you may have tried in the past might have led to food obsession and yo-yo dieting, the Food Foundations (in combination with GLP-1s) help you do the opposite—redirect all that energy, attention, and willpower toward other areas of your life.

3. **Mental Foundations.** This is where we address the behavioral side of weight loss and maintenance, which still needs to be managed while on GLP-1s. We work to surface the negative thoughts and beliefs that may have stymied previous attempts to lose weight, as well as those that are specific to

the use of GLP-1s. This foundation also provides conversational tools to build social support around your GLP-1 journey, so that you can respond to any shamers and critics you encounter along the way. In short, this last piece is designed to help you feel strong, confident, and empowered while using these medications.

## This Book Is for You If . . .

You've read the headlines and heard the gossip about GLP-1s, and you want to separate truth from hype.

You need a safe, nonjudgmental space to consider full-spectrum data about GLP-1s and whether it's something to bring up with your doctor.

You've been prescribed a GLP-1 medication and need a companion plan or more support. Very few doctors have the years of experience that I have treating patients with these meds. Together with my patients, we've learned what works, what doesn't, and how to prepare for each step of the journey.

You're already on your GLP-1 journey and have been hitting stumbling blocks.

And finally, this book is for you if you're interested in any of the following:

A thorough understanding of the science behind obesity and GLP-1 drugs, to help you avoid disease and enjoy a long, healthy life.

Tools to self-advocate at the doctor's office, where old attitudes still rule and many doctors aren't up to speed on medical weight loss options.

Guidelines and recipes that make it easy to eat well while leaving diet culture behind.

First-person success stories from patients who are healthier and happier than ever thanks to GLP-1s, supported by the SoWell Method.

## Freeing the Power of *Your* Will

My patients have as much willpower as anyone else. The greatest tragedy of diet and wellness culture is that it squanders so much of our willpower—scientifically proven to be a limited resource—on often futile or even damaging attempts to lose weight. "Healthy" eating becomes an all-consuming lifestyle, almost a second full-time job.

I grew up in a family of women who struggled with their weight from adolescence to the very end of their lives. My beloved grandmothers were constantly chattering in our kitchen about their next best effort. I heard a lot about "recommitting" after lapses, to whatever the new popular approach might be—whether counting calories, eating grapefruit, or tracking their steps. They tried it all. Meanwhile, as the years passed, they only got heavier, with all the associated health struggles piling on—painful joints, high blood pressure, high blood sugar. Neither of them were ever able to escape the cycle. One eventually died of fatty liver disease, the other from a stroke—both comorbidities of obesity. It's devastating for me to think about how much of their energy went into behaviors that ultimately didn't make them healthier and eroded their self-esteem in the meantime.

A long list of public health benefits will emerge from widespread use of GLP-1 drugs. But one that won't matter to insurance companies or directly impact bottom lines may be among the most important benefits for actual users: GLP-1s give you a viable shot at losing the weight once and then maintaining for life. All that focus and willpower that you once directed at your plate can then be redirected toward what you really care about in life. That's a profound win, and one that I hope everyone reading this gets to experience, wherever your health journey takes you.

# SECTION I

# The Science

CHAPTER 1

# Why "Try Harder" Is Terrible Medical Advice

For centuries, society—including doctors—has heaped shame and scorn on people who carry excess weight. People with obesity are casually, cruelly dismissed as lazy, lacking in self-esteem, weaker, and less competent than their leaner counterparts. There are a lot of ugly reasons for this—racism, classism, and misogyny, to name a few sweeping undercurrents—but because I'm a doctor, this book will focus on the medical story. A primary reason doctors treated obesity as a problem of willpower is that they didn't know any better.

Today, thanks to a quarter century of breakthrough science, we're finally leaving the dark ages of obesity management. The more we've learned about metabolic health, the clearer it has become that many people will never lose significant weight and keep it off through diet and exercise alone—and for others, doing so is theoretically possible but so hard in practice that few will achieve it.

Perhaps you're one of those people: No matter how much you restrict your eating, or count your macronutrients, or increase your exercise, the long-term trend in your weight is up, up, up. The science reveals that it's not your willpower that's failed you—it's your body. Very commonly, chronic overweight is the symptom of an underlying disease. And how do we treat disease, in any other case? Not with shame or exhortations to "try harder," but with medicine.

Think about hypertension, a disorder that can usually be managed with a combination of medication and behavior modification. When the nurse brings out the blood pressure cuff, do you feel your stomach clench, preparing for shame? Does a high reading flood you with negative feelings? For most people, the answer is *no*; your blood pressure is a piece of data, nothing more.

Then, if your blood pressure is high, does your doctor say, "Hmmm—go home, try harder!" Of course not. They likely will offer medications right away to control the symptoms, while also talking to you about lifestyle changes you should make (one of which may be losing weight, since high blood pressure is a comorbidity of obesity).

What makes the experience of these two scenarios so different is that nobody questions the idea that hypertension is a harmful but reversible disease. And until recently, there was no medicine a doctor could offer that would effectively reverse obesity.

## Breakthroughs in Metabolic Health

From decades of research, we now know beyond any doubt that obesity is not caused by weak willpower. It is a chronic, relapsing, and progressive disease with a complex set of causes—so complex that we still don't know everything. Leading scientists and doctors are still hotly debating the root causes of obesity, and not every doctor will agree with my conclusions as an obesity medicine specialist.

Given this complexity, doctors may *never* be able to pinpoint the exact reasons why you or any other specific person became chronically overweight. So that's the first clue that "eat less, move more" or "just try harder" is terrible advice: These are one-size-fits-all directives for an illness that's incredibly individual.

While we still have a lot to learn, we're so much closer than ever before to identifying and treating the root causes of obesity. And while weight stigma is an undeniable problem in medicine, the best way to fight it is to educate yourself about what's happening inside your body, so that you can become your own best advocate and leave shame behind.

With that in mind, congratulations! You've now been accepted into my Mini Obesity Med School. When you finish this section, you will know more than some primary care physicians about metabolic health and the biology of obesity.

## Obesity Medicine 101

Let's start with the old-school, conventional explanations of why people gain weight. These explanations, often together referred to as lifestyle factors, are the origins of "eat less, move more"–style advice:

- **Behavioral:** Some individuals engage in behaviors that lead to overeating and sedentary lifestyles.
- **Environmental:** Changes in the modern world, such as reliance on cars and the prevalence of desk jobs, have led to sedentary lifestyles that promote weight gain.
- **Sociocultural:** Our industrial food culture is making us fat, with many potential culprits: fast food, processed food, seed oils, high-fructose corn syrup, cheap and abundant carbohydrates, lack of access to fruits and vegetables, and more.

Lifestyle factors are important. Just because they're old-school doesn't make them wrong, and I'm not discounting them entirely. Behavioral factors such as unhealthy eating patterns are real causes of obesity and can suggest effective interventions. We also need to work on a societal level to make healthy lifestyles more readily accessible and affordable to all.

But at the same time, these explanations tend to cast obesity as the result of voluntary, and therefore *alterable*, choices, even when knowing that they are strongly influenced by environment and culture. If these were the only culprits, telling someone to "just stop eating" might almost be reasonable.

But thanks to scientific advance, we now have two new root causes to explore and treat: **neurohormonal dysregulation** and **genetics**. They challenge the conventional "eat less, move more" or calories in/calories out approach to weight gain.

---

### DISEASES LINKED TO OBESITY

Before prescribing a GLP-1 medication, your doctor should screen you for the following diseases and disorders. The goal is always to discover and treat the underlying contributors to obesity.

- Polycystic ovary syndrome (PCOS)
- Metabolic syndrome
- Prediabetes
- Type 2 diabetes
- Hypothyroidism
- Binge-eating disorder
- Night eating syndrome
- Sleep apnea
- Depression or mood disorders

---

### Hormones and Your Brain

Science has started to recognize that much of the underlying cause of obesity is physiological, not simply behavioral, due to abnormal neurohormonal signaling within the brain.

To regulate weight, your hypothalamus (in the brain) is in frequent communication with your adipose (fat) hormones, your gut and pancreatic hormones, and the nutrients in the food you eat.[1] When we're in optimal health, all these hormones work together with the brain to maintain energy homeostasis, which means we eat what we need to meet our energy needs, our body metabolizes the food into energy, and our weight stays stable over time. You can't consciously control this hormone signaling, but when it is received in the brain, you feel the effects. These signals control things like how hungry you are, how quickly you feel full, and how good food tastes to you. In other words, this is how the central nervous system compels you to eat, in the same way that your body's need for oxygen compels you to breathe.

When these hormones become dysregulated—and I'll explain some of the reasons that happens in a moment—you can't "will" yourself to stop eating any more than you could will yourself to stop breathing. The problem is physiological, not simply behavioral.

This image might seem complicated, but it's actually a very *simplified* depiction of the complex feedback mechanisms between the brain, the gut, the pancreas, the fat, and your food.[2] It includes the nine weight-involved hormones we know the most about: ghrelin, glucagon-like peptide-1 (GLP-1), peptide YY (PYY), cholecystokinin (CCK), insulin, glucose-dependent insulinotropic polypeptide (GIP), glucagon, amylin, and leptin.

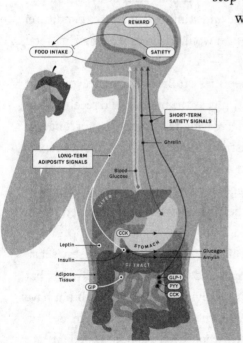

**THE BIOLOGY OF WEIGHT GAIN**

There are more than 400 genes and 40 hormones involved in weight regulation.

## Fat Is an Organ

Few people realize that their fat isn't some passive blob taking up space. In fact, it's a powerful and dynamic organ. I would argue it's the most powerful organ we have. And when it becomes too powerful, it becomes a major driver of the hormone dysregulation that makes it almost impossible to lose weight and increasingly easier to gain it.

Adipose tissue (fat) produces over 600 adipokines, hormonelike substances that are involved in everything from appetite regulation and insulin sensitivity to inflammation and heart disease.[3] One of the most important adipokines is leptin, a satiety hormone that directly communicates with the brain to keep a balance of healthy fat stores. When there is an increase of fat in an optimally lean body, leptin signals the brain to inhibit food intake and stimulate energy expenditure. Conversely, in a too-lean state, leptin would decrease, prompting food intake and conservation of energy.

More fat = more leptin. Since leptin is a fullness hormone, you might assume that this would be a good thing, as the brain would receive a signal to decrease hunger, thereby decreasing fat storage. Unfortunately, you'd be wrong. Like insulin resistance (which we'll talk about next), too much leptin actually leads to a state in which the brain becomes resistant to the hormone's message, leading to reduced satiety, overeating, and weight gain, and furthering the cycling of increased leptin production.[4]

You might think, if you start off lean, shouldn't the body stay sensitive to leptin and maintain its weight and hunger? Historically, yes, but research has shown that the leptin-receiving neurons in the brain have become damaged by the modern Western diet, which has been made "unnaturally" delicious through simple carbohydrates and saturated fat.[5]

Herein lies a difficult cycle to break: Eating hyperpalatable foods impairs brain-leptin signaling, which leads to reduced satiety and increased cravings, which leads to weight gain, which leads to leptin resistance . . . which leads to a desire to eat hyperpalatable foods. (It feels like an evil version of "If you give a mouse a cookie . . .")

### Insulin Resistance

Another form of abnormal neurohormonal signaling results from *insulin resistance*, an extremely common reason people gain weight easily and then have trouble losing it.

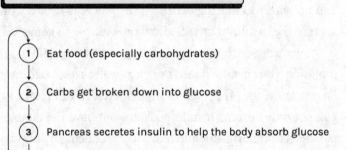

**HOW THE BODY STORES ENERGY**
**(AKA MAKES FAT)**

1. Eat food (especially carbohydrates)
2. Carbs get broken down into glucose
3. Pancreas secretes insulin to help the body absorb glucose
4. Excess glucose is stored as fat
   *Over time, excess glucose and fat cause insulin resistance*
5. Excess fat decreases leptin sensitivity

Food is what our body uses to make and store energy. All food is composed of three macronutrients: carbohydrates, protein, and fat. When you eat food, any food, it eventually gets broken down into building blocks that are useful to your body:

Carbohydrates → Glucose
Protein → Amino acids
Fat → Fatty acids

Glucose, from carbohydrates, is the body's preferred instant energy source. But we can't do anything with glucose alone; it has to be delivered via the hormonal vehicle called *insulin*. Beta cells within your pancreas secrete insulin so that it can be carried off to fuel your brain, your muscles, and everything else.

Your body can do three things with glucose:

- Burn it for instant energy
- Convert it to glycogen in limited amounts for later use
- Store it as fat

What happens when you eat too many carbohydrates and sugar and end up with too much glucose? Your pancreas has to work overtime to secrete the insulin that will allow the glucose to get stored as fat.

Over time, with too much glucose circulating and too much fat accumulating, your insulin doesn't work as well as it used to. You develop *insulin resistance*, the precursor for prediabetes. In full-blown type 2 diabetes, you not only become insulin resistant but have the double whammy of a pancreas that burns out and may stop producing insulin at all.

Once you are insulin resistant, your pancreas continues to pump out the insulin, but your body becomes increasingly desensitized to it. Delivering glucose for energy or storage requires more and more insulin. And while your body and pancreas haggle over how much insulin is needed, the glucose hangs out in your blood, a condition known as *hyperglycemia* (aka high blood sugar).

As insulin levels rise, the body turns up the signals to store fat and increase hunger. Instead of seizing on glucose for instant energy, your body becomes more likely to store it, so you end up with more and more fat. Even in a healthy body, glucose will be stored as fat when your glucose levels exceed your energy needs.

All these hormonal changes caused by insulin resistance explain what's going on behind the scenes when people say, "I'm doing everything and the weight keeps piling on." Doctors used to assume the person was mistaken. In reality, this may be insulin resistance.

In addition to leptin and insulin, a few more key hormonal signals have an important role in the regulation of food intake and energy expenditure via the hypothalamus:

- Ghrelin—secreted by the stomach, stimulates hunger
- Peptide YY (PYY) and cholecystokinin (CCK)—secreted by the intestines, inhibit food intake (decrease appetite), and slow gastric emptying
- Glucagon—secreted by the pancreas, maintains blood glucose and energy homeostasis; in times of limited energy (food) supply, reduces appetite and increases energy expenditure
- Amylin—co-secreted with insulin by the pancreas, suppresses appetite and food intake, slows gastric emptying and suppresses release of glucagon
- Glucagon-like peptide-1 (GLP-1) and glucose-dependent insulinotropic polypeptide (GIP)—secreted by the intestines, stimulates insulin secretion and suppresses glucagon secretion to manage nutrient intake; down regulates hunger, slows gastric emptying

## Why Diets Are Destructive

Weight loss leads to compensatory biological changes that make maintenance almost impossible. Again, hormones are the reason. A 2011 study demonstrated that there are significant hormonal imbalances even up to one year after initial weight loss![6]

In theory, restricting calories should result in fat loss. But I'm sure you've tried this, and you know what happens: Your hunger goes into overdrive. It becomes all-consuming. If you're not actually eating, you're thinking about what you're going to eat next. That's because your gut fires up the hormone ghrelin, which screams, "I'm starving! Feed me!"

We also know that when we restrict calories and lose weight, our body responds by sending less leptin, CCK, PYY, and GLP-1 to the brain—promoting increased hunger and weight regain.

MRI studies have shown that when leptin levels are reduced, the brain responds to the sight of food by firing up its reward centers. MRIs have also shown that each time you diet, these reactions in the brain become more powerful.[7] If you've ever sat at the table unable to stop thinking about the plate of glistening glazed donuts at its center, this is why. You were in the grips of abnormal neurohormonal signaling.

### The Low-Carb "Cure"

Now you understand why your hormones make it close to *physiologically impossible* to exist in a chronically low-calorie state. The more workable way to burn fat is to *decrease your insulin*. Again, in theory, this can be achieved through food restriction alone in the form of a very low-carb, or ketogenic ("keto"), diet.

Just as the nutrients we eat can disrupt proper hormonal function, they can also help heal it. High-sugar, high-carb diets promote insulin resistance. But when you instead *restrict* carbs, there's less glucose coursing through your system and your blood sugar stays low. Your pancreas responds by pumping out less insulin.

When your body needs energy in this glucose-deprived state, it turns to the liver, which stores sugar for exactly this scenario. It's your body's backup generator. You burn through those reserves quickly, in a day or two, and the body moves on to burning fat. This is known as *ketosis*. As you burn fat, your leptin begins to recover, so you're less hungry. And over time, your insulin resistance goes away, too.

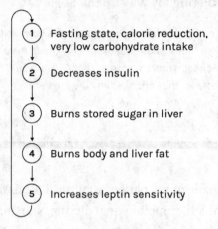

**HOW THE BODY BURNS ENERGY**
(AKA LOSES FAT)

1. Fasting state, calorie reduction, very low carbohydrate intake

2. Decreases insulin

3. Burns stored sugar in liver

4. Burns body and liver fat

5. Increases leptin sensitivity

The problem is that in practice, very few people are able to sustain a low-carb diet long-term. Voluntarily eliminating major food groups isn't what we're designed to do and can have a lot of drawbacks.

Diets don't just fail us, they can make things worse by putting us on the fast track to hormonal dysregulation. No one diets just once—they "yo-yo"—and the more you diet, the harder it is to lose weight the next time. Restriction boosts our hunger signals, so people don't just regain the weight they lost, they put on more. Every diet pushes their set point—the weight that the body tries to protect through homeostasis—a little higher.

I can't tell you how many patients I've seen whose weight problems are the direct result of decades of yo-yo dieting. Gretchen is a stay-at-home mom in the Northeast. (I've changed all the patient names in this book, and sometimes identifying details, to protect their privacy.) In college, at 5 feet 6½ inches tall and 160 pounds, she was unhappy with her weight. Though her body mass index (BMI) put her in the overweight category, she was likely at a metabolically healthy weight. (More about the pros and cons of BMI as a screening tool in chapter 4.)

**My Story: Dieting My Way Up the Scale**

*My entire life, I felt too heavy—not because of how I felt but because of how I looked. Years of dieting eventually made me obese, but I was unwilling to diet anymore. I worried that GLP-1s would be more of the same, but instead, they changed my life forever.*

— Gretchen

As with so many of my patients, cultural ideals around weight and beauty led her to a lifetime of yo-yo dieting, starting in college. Every time she dieted, she lost about 15 pounds and gained back more, and by age 40, she weighed 200 pounds. At that point, she went on one of those "shake" programs, where you drink two shakes a day, furiously exercise, and then have a "sensible" dinner. In five months, she got down to 152 pounds but couldn't sustain it. After that, her weight started to climb, and nothing seemed to be able to stop it. When we had our first meeting, she was 226 pounds, depressed, and angry. She was done with dieting forever—but her history had left its mark. She was insulin resistant, prediabetic, and experiencing debilitating pain in her joints.

### Diets Also Lead to Metabolic Adaptation

It's not only our hunger hormones that lead to weight gain after dieting. Dieting also affects our resting metabolic rate (RMR), the baseline number of calories the body burns just to keep you alive. In short, dieting teaches your body to survive on fewer calories, an effect that persists long after your diet ends, and probably in perpetuity.

This has been shown in a number of studies, but the most famous of them analyzed the RMR of 16 contestants on a TV show from the aughts called *The Biggest Loser*, in which they competed to lose the most body weight in 30 weeks.[8] The bottom line is that metabolic adaptation makes the effort of losing each pound greater and greater the longer you diet.

## Genetics, Epigenetics, and You

There's one final major piece in the puzzle of why excess weight can be so hard to lose: Obesity is overwhelmingly genetic. Studies of twins have shown that familial inheritance accounts for approximately 70 percent of the body's tendency to gain weight. Only 30 percent is tied to environment.[9]

We know this thanks to the pioneering work of Dr. Albert Stunkard, a physician researcher who was among the first to expose deep flaws in medicine's assumption that obesity was primarily a behavioral "disorder of the will," as doctors had described it in the 1800s. The field of obesity medicine might not exist if not for Stunkard's adoption and twin studies in the 1980s.

Stunkard first examined 540 adopted adults and compared their weight to that of their adoptive and biological parents. He found that there was no relationship between the weight of the adoptees and their adoptive parents—the people who had fed them most of their meals and served as role models on their path to adulthood. Instead, their weight closely aligned with that of their biological parents.

These striking findings supported a nature-over-nurture explanation for weight, which was further solidified when Stunkard studied hundreds of pairs of twins who were raised both together and apart.[10] He found that the twins' BMIs were nearly identical, regardless of whether they were raised together or apart, reinforcing the idea that environment (nurture) was largely irrelevant to body weight.

Does this mean we should give up on environmental and behavioral change? Not even Dr. Stunkard thought so. But it does emphasize that weight gain is a largely biological phenomenon, requiring solutions above and beyond individual initiative.

## The Mysterious Obesity Spike

In the years since Stunkard's research, more than 500 genes have been linked to obesity.[11] And yet genetics alone can't explain certain population-level changes in the prevalence of obesity since 1980. Between 1980 and 2018, the percentage of the US population with BMIs over 30 went from 13.4 percent to 42.4 percent. The population with extreme obesity (BMI $\geq$ 40) also increased during this period, from 0.9 percent to 9.2 percent.[12]

So what happened in 1980? Everything from corn subsidies to hyperpalatable junk food to the widespread use of air-conditioning has been suggested to explain the dramatic increase in obesity in the years since. This population-level change is far too rapid to be explained by genetics. However, the emerging science of *epigenetics* provides a possible hereditary component.

Epigenetics, which literally means "on top of genetics," is the study of how genetics and life exposures intersect. These exposures—environmental, nutritional, fetal, viral, and others—all have the potential to change the expression of a gene. As obesity researcher George Bray noted, in a quote made famous by scientist Elizabeth Blackburn, "Genes load the gun and environment pulls the trigger."[13]

The idea that epigenetics might be *inheritable* is still very much up for debate. It might be that whatever new factor that was introduced in 1980 has merely persisted, influencing gene expression in each gen-

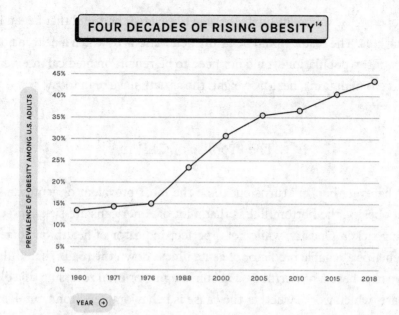

FOUR DECADES OF RISING OBESITY[14]

eration through immediate exposure. In other words, if corn subsidies were the cause of the spike, we've been eating too much corn syrup ever since.

However, some studies have suggested the possibility of inheritable epigenetics of obesity passed down from generation to generation. For example, researchers found that children born to women after bariatric surgery and subsequent weight loss were at lower risk for obesity than siblings born before surgery.[15]

## Why This Matters

Researchers project that by 2030 approximately 50 percent of US adults will have obesity, with as many as 25 percent of adults having severe obesity (a BMI above 35).[16] If we could find a way to combat obesity population-wide in a single generation—a far-reaching but hopeful possibility, if GLP-1s were to become widely accessible and adopted—the hope is that we might finally be able to reverse the trend that began in the '80s. The result would be future generations in which a near majority of the population would not need to be reliant on medical intervention to maintain a healthy weight, the situation we're in today.

## The Promise of GLP-1s

Whatever "bucket" turns out to be the most prevalent or acute cause of obesity, the bottom line is that a lot of Americans are sick and getting sicker. Obesity, while not a perfect indicator of health outcomes, remains a reliable predictor of acute illness down the road. Thankfully, we now have a powerful means of managing or even reversing this disease, which works whether the cause is behavioral, environmental, sociocultural, hormonal, metabolic, or genetic.

# CHAPTER 2

# How GLP-1s Reverse Obesity, End Yo-Yo Dieting, and Protect You from Disease

My patient Amelia is an outgoing, can-do powerhouse who manages a team of nurses in a major US city. She is also far from the stereotype of a person with obesity. She grew up in a family with very healthy habits and was a dancer in high school and college. For most of her adulthood, she worked out seriously, eventually taking up CrossFit and Orangetheory. Her favorite vacation is backpacking through the mountains. And yet when we met in 2020 when she was 34, she weighed 324 pounds.

See if you can identify with how Amelia got there. As an adult, she had hovered between 180 and 200 pounds—but maintaining that weight range had taken a lot of effort. She built a lifestyle around constant dieting and exercise. Even so, in her late twenties, her weight began to creep up. She'd go hard on an eating and exercise program, even hiring trainers and chefs, and lose 40 to 60 pounds—only to gain it back, and more, almost as quickly.

And then the COVID-19 pandemic hit. Amelia was suddenly working eighteen-hour days with no days off. She was emotionally and physically overwhelmed, with no time or energy for exercise. Having started the pandemic at her highest weight ever, she gained about 50 more pounds over a four-month period and watched her health continue to decline.

Her joints hurt so much, it became a struggle to get out of bed some mornings. Meanwhile, her digestive system was a wreck. Any time she ate carbs or sugar, she had terrible stomach pain, diarrhea, and other problems, so she was barely eating. Then there came a devastating point when she realized she wasn't fit enough to go backpacking anymore. At this new weight, she barely recognized herself.

When work-life balance finally returned, she was determined to feel good again. She hired a trainer and ate clean. But after months of working out and eating close to a no-carb diet, she hadn't lost any weight. And she definitely didn't feel any better.

Amelia contacted me at the urging of one of her patients, who had lost more than 100 pounds and overcome binge-eating disorder under my care. At first, Amelia was extremely skeptical about the idea of weight loss drugs. She had all the tools and resources to lose weight and had done it plenty of times before. And yet she knew that this time, there was more going on inside; she was really sick and starting to believe she might need some help.

As always, we started with bloodwork. As a person who had worked hard to be healthy most of her life, it wasn't easy for her to confront the numbers in her labs. She was extremely upset to learn that she had a hemoglobin A1C (HbA1C) of 8.1, confirming type 2 diabetes. She also had high blood pressure and high cholesterol, markers of metabolic dysfunction. Her weight, BMI, and waist circumference put her squarely in the "high-risk obesity" category, a designation that felt shocking.

Amelia's first job as a nurse had been in a bariatric center, so while she well understood that obesity was a disease state, she had been taught that shrinking the stomach through surgery was the most—really, the only—effective intervention. But she also feared the procedure, having seen a small subset of patients experience irreversible damage. She also knew that it wasn't foolproof; in fact, the patient who had recommended me had regained all the weight she'd lost and more after bariatric surgery.

Amelia's interaction with my patient was the first time she had ever heard of GLP-1s. And so my initial step was explaining to Amelia how these new-to-her drugs would not only lead to weight loss, but also reverse the obesity comorbidities she was already suffering from at the young age of 34.

## GLP-1s and the Brain

GLP-1 drugs allow us to manage the hormone dysregulation we discussed in the previous chapter. Remember, these hormones regulate hunger, satiety, and other factors that determine whether the scale moves up or down.

After years of failed attempts to find an effective cure for obesity through hormonal pathways, scientists looking for a diabetes treatment finally produced *semaglutide*—the active ingredient in Ozempic and Wegovy. Semaglutide is a lab-made analogue to the hormone GLP-1. Doctors call it an agonist, or a copy. Mounjaro and Zepbound are also agonists, but of two hormones instead of just GLP-1. This dual agonist, known as *tirzepatide*, comprises GLP-1 linked with a second hormone, GIP.

Some very powerful things happened when researchers flooded the body with long-acting agonists for these hormones, at levels far beyond what nature provides—which is why GLP-1s used in combination with lifestyle changes are now the world's first truly effective protocol for healing the metabolic system and treating obesity long-term.

Let's start with blood sugar.

Lots of people need help managing their blood sugar, not just people with type 2 diabetes like Amelia. Many people who struggle with overweight or obesity are prediabetic, with markers for insulin resistance and blood sugar levels in the high end of the "normal" range. Often their only symptom at this stage is that they struggle harder to lose weight. A shocking study out of the University of North Carolina at Chapel Hill found that only 12.2 percent of American adults are metabolically healthy. Metabolic health was defined as having optimal levels of five factors: blood sugar, triglycerides, high-density lipoprotein cholesterol, blood pressure, and waist circumference, without the need for medications.[1]

Which brings us to **GLP-1's first superpower**: regulating your blood sugar. Data from the SURPASS-1 trial, which studied participants with type 2 diabetes on tirzepatide over 40 weeks of treatment, showed a greater than 2 percentage point reduction in HbA1c for those on the full dose.[2] (The HbA1c test, sometimes referred to as the A1c test, measures the percentage of hemoglobin in your red blood cells that has glucose attached, indicating the average glucose in the blood over the past three months. It is used to diagnose type 2 diabetes and prediabetes.) Almost 90 percent of all study participants achieved an HbA1c of less than 7 percent, the recommended average blood sugar target set by the American Diabetes Association. Of those on the full dose (15 mg), greater than 50 percent achieved an HbA1c of less than 5.7 percent, which is out of the prediabetic range.

How are those results achieved? When blood sugars get too high, the GLP-1 drug talks to the pancreas and says, "Fire up the insulin." It also tells your liver to stop producing sugar. This allows your body to sweep all the extra sugar out of the blood. This reduces inflammation and protects you from a grab bag of health problems.

But even with blood sugar levels in the normal range, you would remain overweight, or gain weight if you ate beyond your energy needs.

Enter **GLP-1's second superpower**: turning the hunger volume down so you naturally eat less. As we've already learned, cutting calories without medication would cause your hormones to scream "eat more!" all day long. But when you take a GLP-1 drug, your stomach holds food longer rather than quickly moving it through to the intestines. A full stomach signals the body to produce less hunger hormones and more fullness hormones. So not only do you get full faster, you stay full longer.

And finally, **GLP-1's third superpower**: talking to the brain *from the gut* to regulate appetite and food intake. The more GLP-1 in the brain, the less hungry you are.

Together, these three superpowers have a profound effect on the communication between the brain, the fat, and the gut. Some other types of weight loss medication act on the brain's reward centers, which compel us to eat. Contrave, which combines an addiction medication with a depression medication, is one example. GLP-1s, meanwhile, don't work on the brain alone. Instead, they fortify the body's built-in back-and-forth system for weight regulation, which depends on the communication loop *between* the brain, the fat, the gut, and the food.

All these factors come together to lower your weight set point *as long as you stay on the drug and continue the lifestyle changes you made while taking it.* And so, for the first time ever, you're able to lose weight and maintain it. It won't be effortless, but you get to stop spending every day of your life fighting your biology, in the gym and at the table.

## Breaking Down the Benefits

Usually information about the benefits of GLP-1s starts with how much weight you can expect to lose. I'm a doctor whose primary interests are prevention and healing, so I'm instead going to start with disease reduction. While so far, the drug is only approved by the Food and Drug Administration (FDA) for diabetes, weight loss, and cardiovascular disease (the latter only when patients are also overweight or obese), people who lose weight on a GLP-1 see improvement or reversal of the following health issues—and this is only a partial list:

- Insulin resistance
- Type 2 diabetes
- Fatty liver syndromes

- Hypertension (aka high blood pressure)
- High cholesterol and heart disease
- Chronic kidney disease (CKD)
- Sleep apnea

The efficacy of GLP-1s for treating type 2 diabetes and its associated conditions is well established, but the first landmark study proving their effect on cardiovascular disease in people without diabetes did not arrive until 2023. In November of that year, Novo Nordisk published full data for its SELECT trial—and it was even better than prevention-oriented doctors like myself had hoped for. Semaglutide in the full 2.4 mg dose was shown to produce the following benefits in obese and overweight people with established cardiovascular disease (CVD) but without diabetes:

- 20 percent reduction in cardiovascular death, heart attack, and stroke
- 18 percent reduction in heart failure
- 19 percent reduction in all-cause mortality
- 75 percent reduction in onset of prediabetes

Lifetime risk of cardiovascular disease in people with obesity, but without diabetes, is about 1 in 2 for women and 2 in 3 for men, so the potential impact of GLP-1 therapy is huge. The data is starting to prove out what I've seen in my practice—that significant excess weight burdens every system of the body. It forces the heart to work harder. Fat in the pancreas, blood vessels, and liver wreaks havoc on the metabolic system. It sets off inflammatory pathways directly linked to 16 types of cancer, prematurely destroys our joints, and damages vessels in the brain, which can lead to dementia—in fact, obesity is now considered the top modifiable risk factor for dementia.[3] Nearly every chronic health condition in the United States is caused, or exacerbated, by excess weight.

The reason GLP-1s are a promising therapy for so many of the illnesses that plague us is simple: They finally **make sustainable weight loss possible.** So many illnesses resolve when patients lose (and keep off) even 5 percent of their body weight.

## What Does It *Feel* Like to Be on a GLP-1?

Media coverage has focused on the unpleasant side effects of GLP-1s—which do exist, and which we'll get into in detail later. Instead, let's start by talking about the most prevalent positives, some of which are surprising.

**Hunger reduction.** The level of hunger reduction varies widely from patient to patient. Almost everyone is less hungry—but most people don't find their hunger has been eliminated completely, despite what you may have read elsewhere, and the effect decreases over time. Which is a good thing! We need hunger cues, just as we need calories and nutrition to fuel our healthy bodies.

**Eating less feels natural.** Perhaps you've heard of the Japanese concept of *hara hachi bu*, in which you stop eating when you're 80 percent full. Popularized by Dan Buettner's Blue Zones diet, it sounds great in theory and is apparently one of the secrets to Okinawans' low calorie intake and resulting longevity. But if you follow the advice, it means you never get to finish a meal feeling completely satisfied—particularly if you're struggling with chronic obesity and have off-the-charts hunger signals. You could say that GLP-1s automate hara hachi bu. People find themselves feeling completely satisfied by a meal that might be 80 percent (or considerably less) of the calories they would have once eaten in a sitting. So despite eating less than they're used to, they're feeling more satisfied—sometimes for the first time in their lives.

**Quieting of food noise.** Liz is a highly successful executive and a mom of two. She recently told me that starting a GLP-1 medication felt like "getting four hours of my day back." For years, she had been constantly obsessing about what to eat next, how to make good choices, and how she should have done better with her last meal. She never thought she could have relief from these pervasive thoughts, and yet it happened even with the lowest dose.

"Food noise"—what Liz described—isn't a medical term; it originates with patients, and you can find it being discussed all over platforms like TikTok and Reddit. While restrictive diets tend to increase food noise for everybody, my patients' experiences strongly suggest there's biology at work as well. For some people, starting a GLP-1 turns off food noise like a light switch. Cravings that had been a constant companion disappear. Previously obsessive thoughts about eating are gone. Like hunger reduction, this effect tends to diminish over time—but the pause gives patients an opportunity to make fundamental shifts in their eating habits and their relationship to food.

**Reduced interest in or outright aversion to alcohol.** Many regular drinkers find they no longer want their nightly glass(es) of wine or beer while taking a GLP-1. This effect is so pronounced that GLP-1s are now being explored as a treatment for alcoholism as well as other addictions.[4] It's worth noting that those who continue drinking often find they're more sensitive to alcohol, with worse hangovers. Much of the horrible feeling you get after drinking too much is due to fluctuations in blood sugar combined with dehydration, two outcomes that can be aggravated while on these meds. So if you do continue drinking, proceed with extreme caution until you know what your system can tolerate.

**Emotional relief from the stigma of excess weight.** This is a big one. No drug can take away all the destructive social messaging that leaves people plotting their self-worth in an inverse relationship with their weight. However, patients experience incredible relief when they see that *reversible biological factors* have led to their being chronically overweight. Obesity stops being an identity and becomes a diagnosis with a doable treatment plan. Successful weight loss, sustained over time, strengthens and solidifies this new outlook.

Amid all this good news, keep in mind that even positive side effects can have surprising ripple effects. For example, when food or alcohol have been a primary source of pleasure, patients sometimes encounter deep feelings of grief or loss, even if they're happy to be meeting their health goals. These feelings shouldn't be ignored or dismissed. There are solutions and supports to manage these ripples, which we'll discuss in chapter 7.

### A PEEK AT AMELIA'S JOURNAL

It took Amelia 14 months, or 60 weeks, to lose 100 pounds—an average of 1.6 pounds per week. But the journey wasn't linear. Some weeks or months there was more weight loss; some weeks there was gain; some were neutral. A major hurdle my patients face is understanding that our weight can be fluid (our bodies are literally made up of about 60 percent fluid, after all) and that the scale doesn't always reward us in the way that we anticipate. Looking back at Amelia's food and lifestyle log, here are a few insights into the toughest parts of her journey:

( 04/12/22 )  *Had first session today, it was a little challenging facing past trauma, I feel triggered. Nervous about weight loss. I am scared to fail. Took Luna to the dog park for a few hours and walked around the lake. (320lbs)*

( 05/10/22 )  *I find that I am not missing carbs or sugar. I wonder how long this will last. I literally am not missing food which makes me wonder if I am eating correctly. Shouldn't I miss something? (299)*

( 09/02/22 )  *Feeling like the weight loss isn't real and am panicked about when it will stop and I will regain. (270)*

( 11/14/22 ) I am just tired and pondering life's greatest questions lol. I am excited for the journey thus far, I am wondering will I forever need medication and will I always need to log. Dr. Sowa says back to the basics with no deviation and she's right but I wonder will I get to an accountable point on my own. (257)

( 12/27/22 ) Processing some of my food choices while at home and trying to process what sustainability will look like once I hit my weight loss goals. (247, 2lbs gained over the Christmas holiday)

( 03/08/23 ) I am adjusting to how I look and feel every day, it's strange. It's as though I find myself trying to forgive myself for the weight gain. Struggling with thoughts around my weight gain, I am having a hard time looking at [old] pictures of myself. (230)

( 09/02/23 ) Comments about my current and previous weight are overwhelming at times. I am tired of deflecting to avoid the comments, people do not realize the impact of their words. (233)

## Emerging Benefits

Currently, the hormone agonist medications on the market are approved by the FDA for the treatment of type 2 diabetes and obesity, as well as cardiovascular disease when patients are also overweight and obese. But research is underway to explore their usage to treat other illnesses. A clinical trial studying the effect of semaglutide on nonalcoholic fatty liver disease (NAFLD) is underway.[5] Eli Lilly has a "tri-agonist" drug (GLP-1 plus GIP and glucagon) in clinical trials that has shown not only a 24.2 percent weight loss over 48 weeks, but also the reversal of NAFLD in 9 out of 10 participants.

The FLOW trial showed that patients with type 2 diabetes and chronic kidney disease who took semaglutide reduced their risk of major kidney disease events by 24 percent, along with significant all-cause mortality reduction.[6]

In a study of people with obesity and sleep apnea, half the participants showed a near remission of symptoms after 52 weeks of treatment with tirzepatide.[7]

While the FDA hasn't yet approved GLP-1s for the treatment of polycystic ovary syndrome (PCOS), I'm one of many doctors who have seen how well it works to relieve the condition. PCOS is a common disorder, affecting up to 12 percent of women of reproductive age, but is a disease state that is often overlooked or minimized at the doctor's office.

PCOS is a chronic condition that causes hormonal imbalances associated with anovulation, irregular periods, infertility, weight gain, insulin resistance, type 2 diabetes, hyperlipidemia, heart disease, hypertension, androgenetic alopecia, and excess facial and body hair. And yet women are often given little guidance when it presents; instead, they're often just put on birth control to help with irregular periods (a common PCOS symptom) and shuttled out the door. Up to 70 percent of these women have concurrent insulin resistance, a precursor for type 2 diabetes and a big driver of weight gain.

When Audrey, age 35, arrived in my office, she had hypothyroidism and PCOS. Like many women with PCOS, she had struggled with her weight for years. When she came to me, she had been trying to get pregnant for more than two years, and was losing hope. Like many with PCOS, Audrey felt stuck and hopeless in a vicious cycle of constant dieting and exercising to maintain her weight of around 190 pounds on her 5-foot-3 frame. When she was first diagnosed by a gynecologist at age 19, she was put on birth control and told PCOS would "likely make it difficult to get pregnant." When she turned 30, being "perfect with her lifestyle" no longer worked, and she slowly crept up to 220 pounds. That's when she started taking Ozempic for rising HbA1c, an average marker of blood sugar. After transitioning to Wegovy, she not only lost 50 pounds, her periods became regular, and likely so did her ovulation. The unimaginable happened—she became pregnant. She has since delivered a healthy baby girl. It is technically recommended to stop a GLP-1 two to three months ahead of planned pregnancy, as there's no data on whether it's safe for pregnancy, but Audrey's is a common story—of losing weight, improving insulin sensitivity, and becoming pregnant without fertility treatment.

Someday, hormone agonists may provide a new line of treatment for dementia, and studies are underway to explore whether these drugs might be effective in slowing or even reversing the course of the disease. Already, a five-year Danish study of people with type 2 diabetes found that those being treated with semaglutide or liraglutide had a lower incidence of dementia.[8]

Given all these health benefits, even some people who don't have BMIs over 30 might find themselves asking, *Should I be on those drugs?* In chapter 4, we'll return to that question.

### My Story: I Got My Life Back

*I'll be honest, the first six months of my journey were so hard. At that time I was so sick that I worried my parents were going to have to prematurely bury their child because of obesity. Then, when I started on Ozempic, my blood sugar quickly went to a normal range. I switched to Mounjaro when my weight loss plateaued. I'll be on it for life. The only time I plan to come off is when I try for my first child, and I'll be working with Dr. Sowa to control my weight with lower carbohydrate eating while having a healthy pregnancy. It's been two and a half years. I've gone* from 324 pounds to 193. It's not the lowest weight I've ever been, but it's a weight I feel good at—and this is the longest I've sustained a weight loss in my adult life. I'm enjoying this new body, this new mind. I just want to see what I can do with it. I'm 36 years old. This is the best I've felt in years. I can run. I don't get winded. I can work out and it's enjoyable.

I still eat lower carb, about 30 to 40 grams a day, but it's because it works best for me. It's a lifestyle choice. My mind doesn't get bogged down, I don't get sluggish after meals, and I have more energy. It's a beautiful thing.

I feel like I have my life back. At the end of 2019, I felt like I physically couldn't handle backpacking anymore. Well, a couple years later when my girlfriend and I checked out venues for our wedding, we went backpacking. We covered about 10 miles a day, in mountainous terrain, carrying 40-pound packs. In five days on the trail, I had zero problems.

My girlfriend is now my wife. Inspired by my journey, she has also lost more than 60 pounds. Instead of constant doctors' appointments and health ailments, I'm able to plan for having children.

— Amelia

# CHAPTER 3

# What the GLP-1 Experience
# Really Feels Like: An FAQ

There's a ton of noise surrounding GLP-1s, both positive and negative. Maybe you heard about the celeb who had to quit because she couldn't stop vomiting, or someone's cousin who lost 30 pounds their first month. Every story is valid, assuming the facts are right. Every experience is unique. The problem is that the extreme cases, good and bad, are the ones that both everyday people and the media most frequently share. These outliers create a distorted view of the average GLP-1 experience.

In this chapter, you'll learn what the science tells us, based on my review of more than 30 clinical trials of liraglutide, semaglutide, and tirzepatide. For questions where there is no data, my answer is based on my clinical experience working with more than a thousand patients.

Again, individual experience will vary. This chapter can't tell you exactly what your GLP-1 journey will look like, but it can tell you what you can likely expect.

## How Much Weight Will I Lose?

How much you'll lose is dependent on a few objective variables, like what your starting weight is, what dosage you take, and whether you have other medical conditions, such as type 2 diabetes.

It's also dependent on one big subjective variable: you. GLP-1 users who make positive lifestyle changes (for example, the SoWell Foundations found in Section II of this book) lose more. But also, some people just lose more naturally. Doctors call them "hyper-responders," and we aren't quite sure why some people have a greater physiological response than others. There's no way yet to predict who will be a hyper-responder and who won't.

But here's what the science from the 68-week trials of tirzepatide and semaglutide say about average losses, measured in percentage of total body weight.[1]

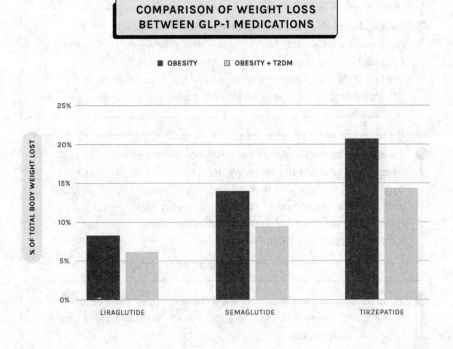

Graph Sources: SCALE trial[2]; SURMOUNT-1[3] and SURMOUNT-2[4]; STEP 1[5] and STEP 2[6]

## Top Takeaways:

✓ **Tirzepatide (Mounjaro and Zepbound)** delivers the best results, with an average loss of more than 20 percent of total body weight. To give you a sense of what that looks like, a 300-pound person loses 60 pounds on average; a 200-pound person loses 40 pounds; a 180-pound person loses 36 pounds.

✓ **GLP-1s are intended to be combined with conscious lifestyle changes.** Both semaglutide and tirzepatide 68-week study participants met regularly with a dietitian to help ensure they maintained a 500-calorie deficit and increased physical activity to 150 minutes a week.

✓ **Women in studies have tended to lose more than men.** In nonmedicated diet and lifestyle interventions for weight loss, women typically underperform compared to men. But in the STEP 1 trial (semaglutide use in people with obesity only), women lost about 18 percent of their total body weight, while men lost 13 percent.

✓ **People with obesity and type 2 diabetes don't lose as much as people who have obesity alone.** We don't know why yet, but some hypothetical explanations include that they have had obesity longer, with increased hypothalamic/hormone dysfunction; that their microbiome has been altered; or that they're on other medications for their illness that promote weight gain.[7]

✓ **The participants were skewed toward the very heavy.** The average starting BMI in these studies was about 38, which is considered class II or severe obesity.

> ✅ **Study participants have been mostly white and female**—more than 70 percent and 80 percent, respectively. We need studies that are more broadly representative of the population.

Here's a graph I love because it shows how effective GLP-1s are compared to earlier weight loss medications. (Metformin regulates blood sugar but has been used off-label for weight loss.)

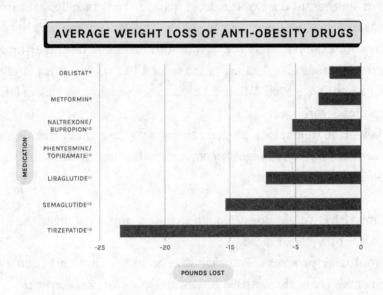

### AVERAGE WEIGHT LOSS OF ANTI-OBESITY DRUGS

The only intervention that still outperforms GLP-1s is bariatric surgery, which reduces the size of the stomach to produce losses averaging 30 to 40 percent of total body weight—but with the considerable downsides of irreversibility and greater risk of complications.[14]

## How Fast Will I Lose?

Many patients mistakenly believe the weight will drop off immediately. But our expectations about total weight loss are based on 68- or 72-week trials. That means it took study participants well over a year to lose their weight. This is not a quick fix!

Healthy and expected weight loss on these drugs is 0.5 to 1 percent of total body weight (TBW) per week. For a 300-pound person, that's up to 3 pounds per week; for a 200-pound person, up to 2 pounds per week.

Also consider that 1 to 2 pounds a week is an *average* loss over time. The actual journey is not so linear, in part because we don't start patients on the full dose of the drug; instead, we titrate up (meaning we increase the dose) over four to six months. Most of my patients on Wegovy, for example, don't see significant weight loss until they move from the initial dose of 0.25 mg to the second (0.5 mg) or third (1 mg) dose. Patients with type 2 diabetes tend to see weight loss kick in later than patients without.

As with all weight loss, progress slows as your weight decreases and 1 percent of your body weight becomes a smaller and smaller number.

So in summary, expect:

- **Slow(ish) weight loss.** Not in a few months, but over the course of a year or more.
- **Nonlinear progress.** You may lose nothing one month, and 8 pounds the next month. Be patient and let the medication work!

## Can This Drug Make Me Skinny?

"Skinny" and "thin" are subjective, but I do get this question a lot and would like to help people set expectations. I have patients who are disappointed that they "only lost 40 pounds" and don't finish their weight loss journey at a size 2 or at their high school weight.

In a tirzepatide study, the average change in BMI was a reduction of 10 points over 88 weeks.[15] Since the average starting BMI was 38, this means participants went from being categorized as severely obese to overweight.

In my practice, very rarely do I see a patient finish with a BMI of 18 to 22, the lowest healthy range, despite the fact that most of my patients combine the medication with significant lifestyle interventions, such as low-carb eating. Many patients achieve a healthy BMI of 23 to 25. Still others settle above 25, technically still overweight according to BMI but with labs that say they're metabolically healthy.

Think about a 180-pound, 5-foot-4 woman with a starting BMI of 30. If she lost the average 20 percent of total body weight after 72 weeks on tirzepatide, her final weight would be 144 pounds with a BMI of 24.7. That's a very healthy, happy weight, but she's still not going to be '90s-runway-model "thin."

My chief goal with patients is a loss of 15 to 20 percent of their total body weight, which allows them to reap all the major health benefits of weight loss. We'll talk more about goal weights in chapter 11.

## Will I Have Horrible Side Effects?

Any kind of extreme reaction is rare.

You are most likely to experience at least one type of *mild to moderate* GI side effect during the titration period. Nausea is the most common side effect, according to some studies, but in my clinical experience, while nausea may be the most frequent, it's constipation or diarrhea that's the most bothersome.

The data supports what I have found clinically: Tirzepatide is generally better tolerated than semaglutide. Nausea is the most dramatic difference: 33.7 percent of users reporting nausea with semaglutide, but only 20 percent with tirzepatide.

I have patients who tell me they've already tried GLP-1s and couldn't tolerate them. But when they try again under my care, following the

Food Foundations in chapter 6 and with targeted supplement support, they do great. The problem wasn't that their bodies were rejecting the meds, but that they didn't know how to avoid the worst side effects with simple changes to their eating and behavioral patterns.

When symptoms do arise, they are almost always easily managed using over-the-counter remedies, although I'll occasionally prescribe medications like a proton pump inhibitor for GERD or Zofran for occasional nausea.

Here's a more specific breakdown of side effects:

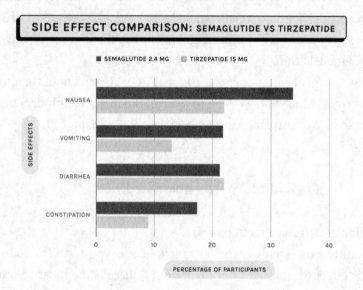

**SIDE EFFECT COMPARISON:** SEMAGLUTIDE VS TIRZEPATIDE

■ SEMAGLUTIDE 2.4 MG    □ TIRZEPATIDE 15 MG

A study participant only had to experience the side effect *one time* in order for it to be counted.

While none of my patients experience every side effect, almost all of them experience at least one. Generally, side effects resolve once their bodies have adjusted to the medication.

"Gastrointestinal adverse events," which were mostly mild to moderate, were reported in 63.5 percent of people taking semaglutide 2.4 mg (the therapeutic dose for weight loss) and 57.5 percent of people taking semaglutide 1.0 mg. But for context, 34.3 percent of the placebo group in that study *also* reported an event.[16]

Across all trials, hardly any patients, typically less than 5 to 10 percent, dropped out due to GI events.[17]

## Does the Medication Become Less Effective Over Time?

Hunger returns, but—and this is a big, important *but*—it doesn't lead to weight regain. In fact, even when their hunger returns, people keep losing.

Somewhere between five months and a year into usage, my patients often report that they feel like the drug (whether semaglutide or tirzepatide) is becoming "less effective." What they're noticing is that their hunger and food noise have started to return. They also might crave a favorite food again, or notice that across the board food has become more desirable.

Their experience reflects what has been seen in research. Participants in a two-year trial of semaglutide were asked about their hunger via a questionnaire at baseline, 20 weeks, 52 weeks, and 104 weeks.[18] At week 20, there was a significant difference between the treatment and placebo groups in feelings of decreased hunger, increased fullness, and ability to resist cravings and control food intake. But by the end of the trial, only a significant difference in the sensation of controlling food intake remained. In other words, the effect on hunger became negligible over time. While at first that sounds disappointing, and sometimes leads some patients to panic, here's what it means: Even though their hunger came back, participants still felt more in control of their eating all the way through to the end of the two-year trial.

The science also tells us that at least through four years—long after the return of hunger—people are maintaining losses far beyond what was achievable in the past through traditional dieting. Weight regain at two years and four years is minimal.[19]

And though it can be scary at first, the return of healthy hunger is actually a good thing. If you use your transition to GLP-1s to build sustainable health, food, and mental foundations, you'll be well equipped to make good choices. Meanwhile, the medication still works in the background, supporting your ongoing metabolic health and weight maintenance.

## Will I Gain Back the Weight If I Stop Taking It?

The short answer is yes. GLP-1s are intended for long-term use. Patients who stop taking semaglutide regain two-thirds of their losses by one year. All cardiometabolic improvements—as measured by blood pressure, lipids, HbA1c, and C-reactive protein—return toward baseline, too.[20]

Additional studies have corroborated these findings. In the Step 4 trial semaglutide users given a placebo after 20 weeks of treatment regained over half their weight at nearly a year.[21] In this study, lifestyle interventions were carried out in both the placebo and medication groups. Everyone in the study had monthly counseling (in person or by telephone), were prescribed a reduced-calorie diet with a 500-calorie daily deficit, and were instructed to increase their physical activity to 150 minutes a week. Even with these continued lifestyle interventions, participants on the placebo could not maintain their losses.

The trend of weight gain was continuing in an upward slope when they stopped the study, suggesting that people would continue to regain. The findings have been the same for tirzepatide.

In the Step 4 study, however, they didn't evaluate intensive, targeted forms of behavioral therapy—for example, a low-carb protocol rather than a general 500-calorie deficit, or strength training versus a general increase in physical activity. Perhaps there is some combination of behavioral interventions that would have been more successful at warding off regain.

Despite the science, I do have patients who have come off GLP-1s and maintained their loss. They tend to fall into three categories: First, younger patients who have the time, focus, and physical ability to commit long-term to a serious exercise program. Second, patients who are willing to prioritize protein and clean eating long-term. And finally, patients who put their excess weight on quickly, for example, after an injury or illness, or because of a medication that induced weight gain, such as steroids or drugs used during IVF.

## What Happens If I Want to Get Pregnant?

According to the package insert, you need to stop taking the medication for two months before attempting to get pregnant and resume only once you're done breastfeeding. There are hardly any studies of pregnant women on GLP-1s, so we don't *know* that it's safe for mother and child. At the same time, what we've seen broadly is that fertility increases while on these medications. A study of liraglutide use among women with PCOS and obesity, for example, showed significantly higher pregnancy rates after 12 weeks on the medication.[22] Informally, positive effects on fertility have been widely reported.[23]

But while many women are getting pregnant on these medications, until there's more science, a doctor can't vouch for their safe use during pregnancy and breastfeeding.

## Will GLP-1s Give Me Gallstones?

No, GLP-1s do not cause gallstones. However, rapid weight loss can—one of many reasons to make sure you're eating enough while on these medications.

First, an anatomy lesson: The gallbladder is a small, hollow organ on the right side of your abdomen, located below your liver. Its job is to store bile, which is used to help in the digestion of fats in the small intestine.

Gallstones form when bile contains too much cholesterol or bilirubin and not enough bile acids or lecithin. And how's this for ironic? Risk of gallstones is increased with obesity, but also with weight loss. (Both states alter the ratio of cholesterol/lecithin/bile in favor of gallstone formation.)

Gallstones are not necessarily problematic. The problem comes if they become too large or get stuck somewhere in the biliary outflow tract. In fact, 10 percent of the population (and up to 30 percent of those with obesity) has gallstones—but only 20 percent of those diagnosed will ever have symptoms or need treatment.

A few factors put people at additional risk:[24]

- Being a woman (a three times greater risk)
- Rapid weight loss (defined as 3 pounds or more a week)
- Significant weight reduction (more than 25 percent of total body weight)

Bariatric surgery patients, who lose weight very rapidly, see an incidence of gallstone formation up to 38 percent.[25] Low-calorie diets alone have been associated with a 25 percent increased risk of gallstone formation.[26] When it comes to GLP-1 use, a large meta-analysis of 76 clinical GLP-1 trials found a small increased risk of gallstone formation, but the overall absolute risk increase was small (an additional 27 cases per 10,000 people treated per year).[27]

Even though GLP-1s do not directly cause gallstone formation, they do lead to weight loss, so I always counsel my patients on what gallstone pain feels like: The pain is located in the upper right part of your abdomen, below the rib cage. (Pain in this area can also be caused by gas or constipation, so if you feel something here, don't panic!) The pain may often come after eating meals, when the gallbladder contracts, and then fade (this is called biliary colic), or be as intense as a constant stabbing (often indicating a full blockage).

Don't ignore symptoms. The waves of pain that come with biliary colic can turn into a more severe blockage—in very rare cases, the stone can get stuck and lead to inflammation in the gallbladder and beyond. If I'm concerned about gallstones, I'll order an ultrasound to evaluate the patient's gallbladder. If the stones are large enough or causing blockage, surgical removal of the gallbladder is the next step.

## Will GLP-1s Give Me Pancreatitis or Pancreatic Cancer?

In 2007, following early case reports of pancreatitis and pancreatic cancer, the FDA issued an alert regarding the potential risk of acute pancreatitis while taking GLP-1s. Due to this concern, GLP-1 receptor agonist product labels warn against their use in patients with a history of pancreatitis.

Pancreatitis is inflammation of the pancreas, while pancreatic cancer is malignant transformation of the subunits of the organ (I often find the two get looped together in this discussion). Pancreatitis can have multiple causes, including gallstones, alcohol abuse, or excess blood triglycerides.

Evaluation of nearly 60,000 GLP-1 users for type 2 diabetes did not find any increased risk of either acute pancreatitis or pancreatic cancer with treatment versus those taking a placebo.[28] As well, a 2024 study of over half a million people found no evidence of increased pancreatic cancer incidence for those on GLP-1 medications.[29] When GLP-1 medications are used for weight loss, specifically, the data is also reassuring: In the two-year semaglutide trial[30] and the tirzepatide trial studying the drug's effect on maintenance,[31] there were no reports of pancreatitis in the treatment groups.

## What About Paralyzed Stomach? Bowel Obstruction?

Gastroparesis, sometimes improperly referred to as stomach paralysis (in which the organ is unable to move food to the digestive tract), and bowel obstruction are extremely rare side effects. A study analyzing 16 million American patients' insurance claim records did find GLP-1s increased the risk of both compared to other weight loss medications—a 4.22 times higher risk for bowel obstruction and 3.67 times for gastroparesis.[32] But the overall risk was still extremely low, and more study is needed.

## Is There a Risk of Increased Suicidality?

This was not found in trials, but after GLP-1s became widely available, there were some reports of suicidal ideation in patients in both the United States and Europe. Regulatory investigations were unable to find a link.

And in fact, a 2024 study of over 240,000 patients in the United States on GLP-1s for overweight or obesity found a *lower* risk of new and recurrent suicidal thoughts than those taking non–GLP agonist medications for weight loss. The findings were replicated among patients taking GLP-1s for type 2 diabetes.[33]

What I notice in my practice is that some patients have relied heavily on food and alcohol to cope with stressful lives. When their desire for these fades away, there's often a transition period in which they find new ways to relax and reward themselves. If patients need help getting over this hump, I refer them to a therapist for extra support.

This is why mood logging is an important part of the SoWell Method—you can watch yourself for patterns and changes, and get help as needed. And as always, if you or someone you know are having any thoughts of suicide, seek help immediately by talking to a mental health professional or calling 988 in the United States.

CHAPTER 4

# Are You a Candidate for a GLP-1?

Just like millions of other people around the world, you no doubt want to know, **"Are GLP-1 drugs right for *me*?"** I'm going to give you the most holistic, honest, hype-free, evidence-backed answer I can provide, because I know how hard that is to come by.

If you're someone who already has a prescription for a drug in the GLP-1 class, *please do not skip this chapter.* There will be moments in your journey when you ask yourself the question again—and what you read here might help you stay the course or prompt a change.

What you read here will still not be a *complete or final* answer. Decisions about managing your health, and especially your weight, are as much personal and emotional as medical. Your body and your health goals are uniquely yours; there's no one-size-fits-all. While a doctor like me can advise you on pros and cons, there is only one expert on *you.*

It's clear that I'm biased. I love to prescribe these meds when a patient's history and labs support it. After studying with Dr. Eric Westman at Duke University, I spent my first years in obesity medicine helping patients lose weight using low-carb and ketogenic diets. Those years were both thrilling and heartbreaking. I remember a patient named Janet, a newlywed who was referred to me as a last stop before bariatric surgery. We were both thrilled when she successfully lost weight—more than 60 pounds on a keto diet—for the first time in many years. Her hunger and cravings were under control and she was making plans to start trying for kids. But as the months passed and her weight loss slowed, she found it increasingly hard to stay on the program. The restrictiveness of the low-carb lifestyle required so much focus that, over time, sticking to it drained her energy and willpower. Attempts to incorporate even healthy carbs, like fruits and whole grains, always seemed to be the gateway to less healthy options. Eventually, she gave up.

In those years, I encountered too many Janets, and that was the heartbreak. Diet and exercise alone were no match for insulin resistance and the other effects of excess weight. I had so many tools to offer, but it still wasn't enough. I often incorporated the older-generation weight loss meds in my treatment plans, but the drugs available then tended to have marginal benefits.

And then came GLP-1s. It was like Dorothy landing in Oz and seeing the world in Technicolor for the first time. Finally, the successes outpaced the heartbreaks by a landslide. My patients met every milestone in their treatment plans, and kept the weight off—not for months, but for years. Without a doubt, they still needed the full tool kit of my program to succeed, but adding GLP-1s was like adding power tools. We could get the job done, reliably, and with relative ease, almost every time.

So yes: The overwhelmingly positive experiences of my patients *have* biased me—except that their experiences also closely match the data from the trials to date. Actually, patients who take GLP-1s while following the SoWell Method tend to outperform the trial data.

Now, on to the $10 billion question: Are these drugs for you?

## If You Think It's a Fad Drug, It's Not for You

"So, about the injectables craze," a doctor said to me the other day, and then posed a completely reasonable medical question. I answered it, but not before I asked her to avoid language like *craze* and *fad* when speaking about GLP-1s. These drugs are neither, and using that language is the wrong way to think about them. It insinuates that they'll be "here today, gone tomorrow," and also that they're poorly researched and probably unhealthy. For anyone considering these medications, this mindset will set you up to fail.

So for starters: These drugs aren't right for you if you're looking for a quick fix. The people who succeed in keeping weight off, with or without GLP-1s, are the ones who make a lifelong commitment to finding and maintaining the weight that supports their peak health, which is different for everyone.

GLP-1s aren't a diet, a fad, or a craze; they are a revolution in healthcare. Much in the way that SSRIs such as Prozac forever changed the landscape of mental healthcare starting in the 1980s and early '90s, these drugs will profoundly change how doctors manage—and how *well* we manage—some of the most common diseases that deprive people of happy, healthy middle age and golden years.

These are the heavy lifters, the power tools, of weight loss. Just like you wouldn't buy a pneumatic nail gun to hang a picture on your wall, not everyone needs these drugs to meet their goals, even within the group that is eligible to use them according to FDA guidelines. For that matter, weight loss itself as a health intervention isn't appropriate for everyone. With all this in mind, let's walk through the conversational steps I take with patients to answer the question together.

## Eligibility According to BMI

The FDA, the agency that regulates prescription medications in the United States, uses BMI to determine eligibility for these meds. The FDA—and with them, your doctor and your insurance company—considers you a candidate if you have:

- **A BMI of more than 30,** *or*
- **A BMI of more than 27,** *if* you also have at least one weight-related comorbidity.

*Comorbidity* means that you have the biomarkers of a weight-related disease such as high blood pressure, type 2 diabetes, or sleep apnea. These are just a few of the over 230 (yes, 230!) medical conditions for which obesity puts you at increased risk.

Every so often, I get an inquiry at my practice that goes something like this: "I'm a personal trainer and lift heavy weights four days a week but still have belly fat. My BMI says I'm overweight. Can you get me injectables?" Already, I know they're probably not a candidate, but I take their height and weight, and quickly calculate their BMI. It's 26—just barely edging into the overweight range (BMI 25–29.9).

At that point, I let the personal trainer know that in my practice, I only accept people with a BMI of more than 27 with a comorbidity or over 30, classifying them as having clinical obesity—meaning they're in the range where their excess weight is strongly statistically likely to impair their health. The personal trainer's weight, on the other hand, is most likely not a health concern. If they persist in worrying, I suggest they visit their primary care physician, who can order labs for a better picture of their underlying metabolic health.

> **My BMI is below 27.**
> **Can I get a GLP-1 for weight loss?**
>
> Sometimes doctors will prescribe these meds even if a patient has a BMI below 27, based on ethnicity or if they're found to have a high fat mass percentage or blood sugar levels indicative of present or future type 2 diabetes.

Are there people with BMIs below 27 who might be good candidates for weight loss medication? Yes. Are there people with BMIs above 30 who might *not* be good candidates? Also yes. But BMIs provide a screening method, a starting point to select for the patients who are most likely to improve their health by losing weight. To put it another way, BMI is how we focus our limited resources on the patients for whom the benefits outweigh the risks and burdens of taking the medication. Only labs can reveal whether your weight is affecting your health, but a screening tool like BMI is a useful starting place.

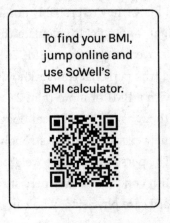

To find your BMI, jump online and use SoWell's BMI calculator.

**SAMPLE BMIs:**

**If a 5-foot-4 woman weighs 157 pounds, she:**

⊕ Has a BMI of 27

⊕ Is considered overweight (BMI 25 to 29.9)

⊕ Is FDA-eligible for weight loss drugs when a comorbidity is present

## If a 5-foot-4 woman weighs 175 pounds, she:

- ⊕ Has a BMI of 30
- ⊕ Is considered obese (BMI 30 or greater)
- ⊕ Is FDA-eligible for weight loss drugs

## If a 5-foot-9 man weighs 183 pounds, he:

- ⊕ Has a BMI of 27
- ⊕ Is considered overweight (BMI 25 to 29.9)
- ⊕ Is FDA-eligible for weight loss drugs when a comorbidity is present

## If a 5-foot-9 man weighs 203 pounds, he:

- ⊕ Has a BMI of 30
- ⊕ Is considered obese
- ⊕ Is FDA-eligible for weight loss drugs

## The BMI Controversy

So what is BMI, really? It's a ratio of weight to height that predicts whether the amount of body fat you have predisposes you to disease.

Many people criticize BMI. They point out that it puts too much focus on the number on the scale instead of on a person's underlying health and is so general that it's not accurate for everybody. They worry that its usage in healthcare can lead people in the direction of dangerous and misplaced obsession with their weight.

They're partly right. At the population level—in other words, looking at grouped data rather than at a specific individual—BMI works great to tell us how weight correlates with obesity comorbidities. Take a look at some of the insights:

---

⊙ Mortality: A BMI in the overweight/class I obesity range reduces life expectancy by 2 to 4 years; a BMI of 40 to 45 reduces it by 8 to 10 years (similar to smoking!).

⊙ Stroke: For every 1 unit increase in BMI, risk increases by 4%.

⊙ Type 2 diabetes: Eighty percent of cases are directly related to obesity.

⊙ Heart failure: Risk increases twofold with a BMI greater than 30.

---

However, at the individual level—you, sitting with your doctor—BMI's prediction accuracy can break down. People who have a lot of muscle mass, like the trainer in the earlier example, also have high BMIs, because muscle is heavy. (Note: If you're sedentary or just an average exerciser, you're probably not in this category.) Postmenopausal women can also be misclassified by BMI, because of normal, hormone-related shifts in the ratio of muscle mass to fat mass. BMI doesn't distinguish between men and women or tell us anything about the role a person's race or ethnicity is playing in their weight or predisposition to disease. Population studies have helped us learn that Asians have higher weight-related disease risks at lower BMIs. China and Japan define overweight as a BMI of 24 or higher and obesity as a BMI of 28 or higher; in India, overweight is defined as a BMI of 23 or higher and obesity as a BMI of 27 or higher.[1]

That's why BMI is only a starting place, not an ending place, to think about your personal health goals. All it can tell you is that you *might* have more body fat than is healthy.

Doctors will also use waist circumference and body fat measuring devices to get more specific insight into the actual amount of fat in your body.

Waist measurement as an indicator of obesity varies by sex and race. A person is considered to have obesity if their waist measurement is:

- ≥40 inches for men (African American, Caucasian)
- ≥35 inches for women

The International Diabetes Federation has defined different cutoff points for different ethnic groups, with Hispanic and Asian populations having an obesity cutoff 3 to 4 inches lower than their Caucasian counterparts.

More advanced tools, like DEXA scans and body composition scales, and less fancy ones, like skin calipers, can also help define obesity. (More on this in chapter 10.) Women with more than 30 percent body fat and men with more than 25 percent body fat are considered to have obesity.

But measuring your body fat, even accurately, doesn't provide a complete answer to whether you should lose weight. It's still only part of the conversation.

## How to measure your waist circumference

Stand and place a measuring tape around your middle, just above your hip bones. Make sure tape is horizontal around your waist, and keep the tape snug around your waist, but not compressing the skin.

Measure your waist just after you breathe out.

For a printable measuring tape, scan the code:

> ### THE
> # Disappearing Obesity Paradox
>
> Fat in itself isn't bad. It can protect us from falls, keep us warm, and support us when we're sick and can't eat. But the idea that it protects us from disease—once popularly known as the "obesity paradox"—has long been considered false.

## Is Your Excess Weight Affecting Your Health?

A lot of the cultural chatter around GLP-1s associates their runaway success with our society's obsession with skinniness. The obsession is real, without a doubt—but for most of the folks that end up in my office, "skinniness" isn't the goal. Many people I work with have real ambivalence about losing weight. They have been at a weight society deems "too big" their entire lives—and though they've struggled, most of them have come through it with healthy self-esteem. Their size and their lifestyle are part of who they are, and the idea of changing either brings grief.

Take my patient Scott. Food was a big part of his identity. He was a proud foodie who liked to celebrate life with lavish meals and good wine, which he collected. He had been overweight since childhood, and now that he was in his forties, the problems were stacking up. Nearing 300 pounds, he had labs showing high blood sugar and elevated liver enzymes—neither high enough to label him "diseased," but getting close. Worse, on a lot of days, he just didn't feel good anymore.

When I first met Scott, he hated the idea of being on a medication for life—especially a GLP-1, which he saw as the end of his life as a bon vivant. Losing weight wasn't just a doctor's order, it was a small identity crisis. He tried to lose weight with a low-carb diet, but every weekend became a bender. He started on metformin for his blood sugar, and tried the weight loss drug Contrave, which can help people overcome cravings. But he couldn't stop "falling off the wagon," as he put it.

Many patients, like Scott, may have had points in their lives when they were pursuing weight loss for vanity or to meet a social ideal, but when they come to me, it's because they're scared for their health. They usually have some kind of significant problem that is likely to be relieved if they can lose even 10 percent of their body weight. Their goal is not "I want a bikini body." Their goals are things that I bet you identify with:

"I want to be here to meet my grandkids."

"I have small children and/or aging parents and need enough energy to take care of them."

"I need to keep my brain sharp for work."

"I want to be able to enjoy my favorite physical activities, without pain."

The question every patient has to answer, with the best available data and with their gut, is this: *Is my excess weight affecting my quality of life or putting me in danger?* What makes this particularly tricky is that "danger" is subjective and dynamic. Each person has to define what's acceptable for themselves, and what trade-offs they're willing to make to be "safer" now or in the future—and those assessments may change over time. For example, you might have smoked when you were twenty, only to be horrified by cigarettes when you were forty. Motorcycles represent freedom and fun to some, and death machines to others. Some people live for today, others plan for tomorrow. You get the idea.

*If health problems related to excess weight are affecting your quality of life or putting you in danger, a GLP-1 may be right for you.*

For Scott, the answer became *yes* after the pandemic lockdowns in 2021. He had reached his highest weight of 306 pounds, had just been diagnosed with type 2 diabetes, and had all five markers for metabolic syndrome (more on what this means below). He started Ozempic, along with a low-carb diet, and when Mounjaro became available, switched to that. Two years later, he was maintaining at 226 pounds, and his diabetes was in full remission.

Is Scott still a foodie? Using a GLP-1—as well as experiencing the health problems that led him to treatment—has undoubtedly changed his relationship with food. It's no longer the center of his universe. But what the old Scott didn't expect is that the new Scott enjoys life as much as ever. It turns out it's easier to be a bon vivant when you're feeling great. He's also thrown himself into his other longtime passion, flying small planes.

### *Why Your Labs Matter More Than Your Weight*

Again, BMIs are only a screening tool, and weight itself isn't always a health problem. Peter Attia, in his bestselling book *Outlive: The Science and Art of Longevity*, puts it well: "Obesity is merely one symptom of an underlying metabolic derangement, such as hyperinsulinemia, that also happens to cause us to gain weight. But not everyone who is obese is metabolically unhealthy, and not everyone who is metabolically unhealthy is obese."

My only quibble is that, as we've discussed, fat is a dynamic organ. In my medical opinion, excess fat is both a *symptom* of metabolic issues and a *cause* of hormonal dysregulation and myriad other negative health effects. That said, Attia's point is crucial: The five markers of *metabolic health* tell you much more about your individual health than the number on the scale or your BMI.

Metabolic syndrome is defined as having at least three of the below markers, but the more of these criteria you meet, the more likely you are to have insulin resistance that is thwarting your efforts to lose weight—and the more likely you are to experience cardiovascular disease, like a heart attack or a stroke. True metabolic health is the absence of *any* of these markers:

1. High blood pressure (>130/85)
2. High triglycerides (>150 mg/dL)
3. Low HDL cholesterol (<40 mg/dL in men or <50 mg/dL in women)
4. Central adiposity (waist circumference >40 inches in men or >35 in women)
5. Elevated fasting glucose (>110 mg/dL)

Metabolic dysfunction is only one of a raft of weight-related health issues that lead people to make losing weight a health goal. Below are some of the most common health issues revealed by lab work that lead my patients to try GLP-1s:

- Insulin resistance or type 2 diabetes
- Hyperlipidemia
- PCOS
- Nonalcoholic fatty liver disease

Outside of labs, many of my patients are dealing with:

- Joint and back pain
- Sleep apnea
- Weight gain caused by medication
- Weight gain during or leading to menopause
- Fatigue

## Don't Expect "GLP-1 and Done"

Finally, strong candidates for these drugs understand that there's no such thing as "GLP-1 and done." The people who I see succeeding long-term on these meds understand that they're not a cheat or a fast pass, no matter what ignorant, fatphobic people might have to say about it. **You still have to do the work to change your underlying habits and thought patterns related to food and weight.** The drug only provides a window in which making these changes is easier and more effective long-term, because the medication normalizes the underlying hormonal dysfunction. GLP-1s will almost guarantee you'll lose weight, but only by using them in partnership with lifestyle changes will you maintain the loss long-term.

As well, weight gain isn't *only* caused by metabolic disorder. GLP-1s are often a first step, not a complete treatment. Part of the journey is evaluating for other factors that might be making someone overweight, such as:

- Sleep apnea (this one is a bit chicken-and-the-egg, but low-quality sleep has a major effect on weight)
- Mental health issues
- Emotional eating
- Autoimmune diseases like lupus or rheumatoid arthritis, which can significantly impair physical activity
- Thyroid diseases like Hashimoto's
- Vitamin deficiencies—for example, low iron, vitamin D, or vitamin B12 may be making you feel sluggish or unwell, leading indirectly to weight gain
- Medications that cause weight gain, such as steroids, SSRIs, or post-cancer treatments

Many physical and emotional factors contribute to your weight and health—and GLP-1s are only one part of a broader journey toward better health.

## GLP-1 Drugs Aren't for Everyone

The FDA guidelines for these drugs specify that they are for "chronic weight management." A less formal way to put this is: These drugs are for people who have tried everything else and need help to avoid chronic illness related to their weight.

Not everybody needs GLP-1s, and not everybody needs obesity medicine. Think of it like therapy. I think about a patient I worked with named Mary. She wanted to join my SoWell Virtual Weight Clinic, but only had about 10 pounds to lose. I almost turned her away because her BMI was borderline healthy; still, she felt she needed help, so I listened. She told me was in a really stressful period of her life, taking care of ailing parents and young kids at the same time. Even though she had only gained 10 pounds, she felt that something in her health wasn't right.

It turned out a couple of things were going on. First, her labs did show signs of early insulin resistance; if her weight continued to climb she'd probably be back in ten years needing to be treated for type 2 diabetes. But the more immediate cause of her weight gain was her mental health. Her caregiving responsibilities, helping two aging parents with debilitating health circumstances, had left her more stressed than she'd been in her entire life. She knew this, but didn't realize it had any connection to her eating until she began tracking her emotions on her food log as part of SoWell's Habit Foundations. She noticed that after challenging caregiving moments—for example, a painful encounter with her mother's faltering memory—she would eat something like a cupcake. For months, she had been using junk food as a coping mechanism, far outside her usual MO before the upheaval in her family life.

Mary did not need a GLP-1, but she was a great fit for a weight loss medication called Contrave. This drug—a combination of the antidepressant bupropion and the anti-addiction medication naltrexone—gave her just enough of a boost in emotional regulation that she was able to find healthier ways to cope with her stress. The medicine she needed was one to support her mental health, not her metabolic system. She also needed some habit changes, and started incorporating a daily walk for relaxation and stress relief. These walks also gave her time to process some of the emotions she was having around the situation with her parents. She quickly took off the 10 pounds, and her labs three months later showed that all the indicators of metabolic health were back within normal ranges.

What I'd like you to take away is that obesity medicine, along with the SoWell Method, offers a full, wide-ranging tool kit for managing weight. If you don't qualify for GLP-1s or can't get access to them, you still have many options and avenues to improve your health.

# The SoWell Method for Sustainable Success on GLP-1s

CHAPTER 5

# The Habit Foundations

Does even the sight of a scale bring up emotions for you? You're not alone. Many patients in my program are alarmed when they first learn that a daily weigh-in is a recommended part of the SoWell Method. When my patient Grace heard this, she almost quit.

Grace had thrown out her home scale years ago because weighing herself was so triggering, dating back to a traumatic experience in middle school. As she recalls, all the girls in her class were forced to line up in the hallway. A nurse then weighed them, one by one, without any privacy. Grace had always felt she was heavy. The shame of that moment was seared into her memory: standing on the medical scale while the nurse slowly moved the weights into balance, feeling like every eye in the room was locked on the numbers. When the nurse finally moved her along, she ran to the bathroom, locked herself in a stall, and burst into tears.

Regular weigh-ins are important for anyone who wants to lose weight and keep it off. They are among a handful of **small but impactful habits** that have been proven to support healthy weight maintenance long-term. Unfortunately, few people build these habits, for the same reason that Grace had avoided the scale: They trigger all the hurtful emotional baggage that we have accumulated from living in a society where people—in the media, for sure, but sometimes even our friends and families—equate our weight and what we eat with our character and self-worth.

And yet these habits are important to our health. Having helped people lose thousands and thousands of pounds, what I've found is that the patients who are the most successful—defined by me as 15 percent or greater total body weight loss *maintained long-term*—are those who embrace the SoWell Habit Foundations and make them stick.

Our goal in this chapter is to start that process, and to do it in a way that moves you toward **emotional neutrality** about your weight and the process of losing it. Emotional neutrality means feeling the same way you do about your scale as you feel about your toothbrush: *emotionless.*

That brush is a neat little tool for keeping your teeth clean; nothing more, nothing less. Sometime, long ago, you built the habit of using it twice daily. These days you barely think about it, even when the brush is in your mouth. You just do it, and then return to your day, enjoying your minty-fresh breath and the knowledge that you're doing what you can to avoid cavities.

At the beginning of your journey, it may be hard to imagine you'll ever feel that way about the habits introduced in this chapter. **You will get there.** One of the beautiful things about GLP-1s is that they quickly and dramatically shift how we experience food and our bodies. Longtime assumptions about "the way things are" and "the way they have to be" are suddenly disproven. This creates a window of opportunity to make deeper, more lasting changes. We can look at old patterns with curiosity instead of anxiety, and replace them with updated routines that better support our health.

I've seen hundreds of patients grow into emotional neutrality. It doesn't happen right away, but if they trust the process, they get there. Grace, for example, is now comfortable with her scale for the first time in her life. It's not because she likes the numbers better (although she *is* at a healthy weight now), but because that tiny little habit, maintained over time, now leads to *less anxiety* and *more comfort*—a scenario that once seemed impossible to her.

## The Why Is the Way

Before we dive into our Habit Foundations, we need to unlock the secret to making habits stick. Let's think about toothbrushing again. Building that habit takes time and patience. I've been helping my son make it a habit for almost ten years and he *still* needs a reminder many—OK, most!—days.

We've been able to keep at it so long for a very simple reason: There's a clear *why*. We don't want cavities! And there's even a short-term perk: It's nice to feel clean and fresh.

Now shift that thinking to weight loss. Take my patient Meghan, who gained weight rapidly during college after she quit dancing, the central focus of her teenage life. When she was in her early twenties, she had bariatric surgery. She very quickly lost 100 pounds—and then gained it all back, plus a few more pounds, over the course of two years.

At age 34, she did the SoWell Method with the support of Wegovy. Three years later, she has maintained a 125-pound weight loss and is doing great. "I'm completely confident I'll maintain this weight for life," she told me—a huge transformation, given that after her big regain before, she was terrified she could never maintain.

The biggest difference between Meghan's two experiences and their outcomes wasn't bariatric surgery versus the meds. **It was learning her why.** The first time she lost weight, she did it because her doctor recommended it and because she missed her dancer's body. The second time, she wanted to lose weight because she had learned she had all five markers of metabolic syndrome. Her father had recently passed, and her aging mother was increasingly dependent on her for help. She was in a new phase of life, and she was scared for her long-term health. When she started, we didn't just talk about her *whys*—we wrote them down, and so should you.

Meghan's *whys*:

- I want to reverse the indicators of metabolic syndrome so that diabetes won't be my future.
- I want to have the strength and stability to be able to take care of my mom.
- I want to be energized and clearheaded for work.

---

### IDENTIFY YOUR WHYS

(1)   Only include one related to weight, appearance, or fashion.

(2)   Write them down.

(3)   Keep them visible.

---

It's crucial that only one of your whys be related to vanity or appearance—reasons like, "I want to fit back into my favorite clothes" or "I want to be a size 10 by my daughter's wedding."

I said this earlier, but it's worth repeating: **Skinny isn't motivating long-term.** The kind of whys that make habits stick are the ones rooted in health or that support a goal that's much bigger than yourself, like Meghan's wish to be a good long-term caregiver for her mother.

For one of my favorite patients, Janelle, *skinny* wasn't just a weak motivator, it was actually a *de-motivator.* Janelle had been overweight her whole life, but really liked her body. Her adult weight had cycled between 220 and 280 pounds, even though she was an active and enthusiastic water aerobics instructor. Being big and healthy was her brand—until she started having some serious health problems related to her weight in her forties. Her blood pressure was very high, she was prediabetic, and she had a family history of both stroke and type 2 diabetes.

She cared about her health, but the prospect of weight loss scared her. She thought she might lose herself if she got too small. "That's not who I am," she told me. I assured her that even losing 10 to 15 percent of her current weight—25 to 40 pounds—would likely improve her current health problems. A low BMI did not need to be the goal. Janelle didn't have any "vanity" whys. She wanted to have more energy, resolve her concerning health indicators, and take the steps that would improve her chances to enjoy a long, healthy life.

Every time she lost 10 pounds, Janelle and I would have a check-in. "Janelle, do you feel good?" I'd ask her. "I feel really good," she'd answer. "OK, great. And do you also still feel like yourself?" So far, the answer has always been yes, and we'll keep on asking the question.

Recently she hit 40 pounds down, and she feels so good, she wants to lose 10 pounds more. Her last labs showed a huge improvement in her blood sugar, and her blood pressure is approaching normal.

As time passes, the goals you write down will serve you in a second way: as a valuable track record of your success. Once you've achieved a goal, it becomes very easy to take your new state of health for granted. For example, one patient had the goal to not get winded while walking up subway steps. One year later, she was lifting in the gym twice a week and working on new goals. Anytime she struggled, she'd pull up her original goals and get a big boost from seeing the proof of how far she had come.

## Habit Foundation 1:
### Record Your Weight *at Least* Once a Week

Mr. Rogers, the beloved children's TV host, was a very lean man. He stayed that way by stepping on the scale every day. If he was down a pound, the story goes, he ate a cookie for dessert. And if he was up a pound, he did an extra lap on his daily swim. Despite having been an overweight child, his daily habit provided a system of checks and balances that allowed him to stay trim until his death at age 74. His weight was simple data used to inform his next steps—and that's what I hope it becomes for you, too.

Diet culture run amok has turned bathroom scales into public enemy number one. But we need to heal the insanity, not throw out the tool that supports one of the cheapest, easiest, fastest habits there is to maintain your health. The National Weight Control Registry tracks the "unicorns" of the pre-GLP-1 weight loss world, those people who have maintained weight loss for an average of 5.5 years. Seventy-five percent of members in the registry weigh themselves at least once a week.

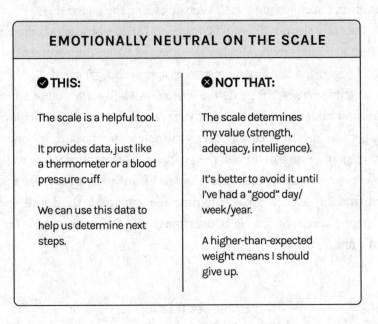

### EMOTIONALLY NEUTRAL ON THE SCALE

| ✅ THIS: | ❌ NOT THAT: |
| --- | --- |
| The scale is a helpful tool. | The scale determines my value (strength, adequacy, intelligence). |
| It provides data, just like a thermometer or a blood pressure cuff. | It's better to avoid it until I've had a "good" day/week/year. |
| We can use this data to help us determine next steps. | A higher-than-expected weight means I should give up. |

## Why I Recommend a Daily Weigh-In

The reason to weigh yourself daily isn't so that, like Mr. Rogers, you can respond to any variation with an immediate change in your behavior. For most people, especially women, that would put you on some kind of wild roller coaster. Our daily weight is extremely fluid—because *we* are extremely fluid, with about 60 percent of our body weight being water.

On a daily basis, I want you to **weigh in, record your weight, and move on**. The value is in the aggregated data, used to suggest changes we need to make over time. And over time, as you see that number go up and down daily, you build trust that the process works, despite fluctuations. It's also a habit that acts as a daily affirmation of our commitment to healthy new behaviors. You can do it right after you brush your teeth in the morning—just another daily feel-good routine.

That's the goal, OK? It may not be your starting place, and that's all right. Foundational habits are a work in progress that get easier over time. If you know that you're not ready for a daily weigh-in, commit instead to a weekly one. **Pick a day and stick to it.** Don't negotiate with yourself. If you pick Sunday, that's your day—even if Saturday you went to a wedding and toasted with champagne and ate salty food and a big slice of cake. It doesn't matter what the scale says; all that's important is that you record the data.

Another reason I recommend a daily weigh-in, when you're ready, is that many patients are surprised to find that the frequency actually helps *support* the goal of emotional neutrality. When you wait a week or more between weigh-ins, the fear can build up, leading to anxiety and more and more time between scale visits. Before you know it, the scale is back in the closet, gathering dust.

Weigh yourself:

- No more than once per day
- No less than once per week
- Indefinitely into the future

Indefinitely means . . . forever. Even when you really don't want to. Weighing in may be more important to maintenance than it is to losing. My patients who have kept their losses off for more than five years are still **weighing in daily**. They might lapse for a day or two, but then they're back on the scale. It's their friendly reminder of their healthy lifestyle. You'd never quit brushing your teeth, right?

### *What About Travel?*

I recommend that all my patients who travel more than once or twice a year get a travel scale. Often a trip that starts as a seven-day break from the scale becomes an *indefinite* one: You come home and don't want to see a "shocking" number, so you decide to "get back on track" before you weigh in. You wait a week, and then another week, and then another . . . You get the picture.

My patient Beth does marketing for a major sports association, a job that takes her all around the world—always with her travel scale.

**My Story: The Travel Weigh In**

*At first I thought Dr. Sowa was insane with this travel scale business. But now I find comfort in the routine and I don't have to face the scaries when I get home. I was nervous that with the travel building new habits would be impossible, but I also knew the timing would never be perfect. I'm glad I didn't wait, because it's working!*

**— Beth, 42, down 30 pounds on
Zepbound in her first three months**

### Habit Foundation 2: The Food Log

Food logging in the SoWell Method isn't like using MyFitnessPal or a diet app. You're not counting calories, or even macros. You're actually going to log a few things: what you ate and when, how hungry you were, and what mood you were in.

And you're *definitely* not stressing about your log. The goal is to eat as usual, and record your choices and the circumstances around them without judgment. Missing a day or a meal isn't a sign that you're bad, or careless, or not meant for this journey. It's a sign that you're a human being adopting a new habit.

## Start Logging Today

If you use the digital version, store it wherever it's most accessible—on your phone, tablet, or computer. Then, create a daily alarm to remind you to log. The best time to log is right after you eat—most people have terrible food recall, and by the time 24 hours have passed, they have no idea what they ate the day before.

Make it as easy and convenient to log as you can. Grab our digital template or download a copy to print out here:

## HOW TO KEEP A NEUTRAL FOOD LOG

**✓ THIS:**

The log is a helpful tool that provides data.

It provides data, just like a thermometer or a blood pressure cuff.

We can use this data to help us determine next steps.

**✕ NOT THAT:**

My food log determines my value (strength/adequacy/intelligence).

It's better to avoid it until I've had a "good" day/week/year.

A worse than expected meal/day/week means I should give up on my goal.

*When to Start Logging*

Many of my patients say, "I'll start logging when the medication starts working and I have things under control." In fact, the ideal time to start your food log is **two weeks before you make any other changes**, including taking your first dose of medication. That's why it's right up here in chapter 5, before the Food Foundations, and before the chapter on starting your meds. (Note that I say this is the *ideal* time to start, but you'll benefit from the Habit Foundations no matter where you are in your GLP-1 journey.) Food logging will be very important throughout the period when you're losing and for about six months into maintenance.

In these first two weeks, filling out the food log provides you with a baseline. It's a chance to identify patterns in your eating *before* you're on the meds. Also keep in mind that when take your first dose, you may not feel that well. It's so much easier to lay the groundwork for a new habit now, when you're feeling strong.

Let's go through the log piece by piece, so you understand *why* you're doing it (always important!) and what to take away.

*"What I Ate/Drank"*

By tracking your eating *before* you start the meds, you'll learn how your choices today compare to the Food Foundations you'll be moving toward in chapter 6. This is important, because you can plan for the likely changes you'll make to avoid side effects once you start your meds. For example, you might learn that you're only eating protein at dinner and not drinking any water—both habits that could lead to unpleasant outcomes.

I had one patient who was a big snacker. She loved the "healthy" snacks: the skinny popcorn, the low-sugar chocolate, the 100-calorie

**SNAPSHOT #1**

| TIME | WHAT I ATE/DRANK | NOTES (MOOD, CIRCUMSTANCES, ETC) |
|---|---|---|
| 9:00AM | Cold brew with scoop of protein powder | |
| 12:00PM | Egg salad over chopped lettuce and tomato | |
| 3:00PM | Cucumbers and hummus | |
| 6:00PM | Shredded chicken, roasted veggies and ⅓ cup quinoa | Glad I had planned this, was hungry after my workout and thought about doing the drive-thru instead! |

**SNAPSHOT #2**

| TIME | WHAT I ATE/DRANK | NOTES (MOOD, CIRCUMSTANCES, ETC) |
|---|---|---|
| 8:00PM | Linguine and shrimp, 2 glasses of white wine | Work dinner, and there weren't great options - tried my best. |
| 7:00AM | Electrolytes, no coffee | Took my shot yesterday morning + combo of carb-heavy work dinner led me to feeling nauseous this morning. I shouldn't have had wine with the pasta. |
| 10:00AM | Sipped a protein shake | |
| 5:30PM | BBQ chicken with a few bites of broccoli and potatoes | |
| 5:30PM | Cheese stick + more electrolyte water | Starting to feel better. |

💡 Identifying patterns in the side effects will give you the data you need to troubleshoot and feel better.

**SNAPSHOT #3**

| TIME | WHAT I ATE/DRANK | NOTES (MOOD, CIRCUMSTANCES, ETC) |
|---|---|---|
| 7:00PM | Coffee with chia seed pudding and an apple | |
| 10:00AM | French toast and bacon + mimosa | Out to brunch - wasn't planning on this meal, but loved it |
| 2:00PM | Ice cream cone | After brunch stroll with friend, ate half - didn't really want, but friend did. A little overstuffed. |
| 5:30PM | Electrolyte water | |
| 7:00PM | Peanut ginger salmon + cucumber smash | Back to regular programming! |
| 9:00PM | Fiber | Feeling a little, ahem, irregular today |

💡 The log won't be useful if all you log are "healthy" choices. There are no bad foods, and logging them can help provide important information about why you have a craving.

packs. Even though she was eating all the time, she ate hardly any protein—which is key to getting the nutritional density you'll need on a GLP-1. Once she learned the Food Foundations, she could see that she'd be better off swapping some of her popcorn for protein-rich snacks and meals.

Remember to stay neutral! This is only data. Avoid the compulsion to change what you eat to match what you think you *should* eat—or to self-edit when you track your foods. The goal is an honest readout. Be as specific as you can, but don't feel like you need to haul out the measuring cups.

## "Hunger Scale"

Here you'll track your level of hunger before *and* after you eat, on a scale from 1 to 10. As we discussed in chapter 1, one of the side effects of metabolic syndrome and chronic overeating is that our hunger and satiety signals, controlled by hormones, often go haywire. Some people may experience more hunger overall and lose the ability to feel satisfied once they're eating. Others eat compulsively, and never allow themselves to get hungry. Either way, the result is that we stop paying close attention to how we feel when we eat. Instead of satiety, your cue to stop becomes the feeling that you're physically stuffed, even to the point of discomfort.

GLP-1s provide a unique opportunity to become more aware of your hunger signals. By learning to check in with your hunger and fullness in these early weeks, you're preparing yourself to practice mindful eating—first during the dramatic shift when you start medication, and then long-term, when healthy hunger signals return and provide important cues to guide both what you eat and how much.

It's also important to stay on top of your hunger between meals. If you let yourself get too hungry, it can lead to poor choices when you do finally sit down to eat.

**THE HUNGER/FULLNESS SCALE[1]**

(1) So hungry you are weak.

(2) Very hungry. Irritable, low energy, large amounts of stomach grumbling, food thoughts every few seconds.

(3) Pretty hungry. Stomach is beginning to growl. Thinking about food every few minutes.

(4) Beginning to feel hungry and have thoughts about food.

(5) Satisfied; neither hungry nor full.

(6) Slightly full or pleasantly full. (Stay within this zone for the best hunger control.)

(7) Slightly uncomfortable; could have stopped eating several bites ago.

(8) Feeling stuffed and uncomfortable.

(9) Very uncomfortable; stomach aches or is distended.

(10) So full you feel sick.

## *"Notes (Mood, Circumstances, Etc.)"*

Logging the *circumstances* (or what cognitive behavioral therapists call "events," more on this in Chapter 7) around our eating helps reveal the hidden influences behind our food choices—especially our moods and emotions. Biology is a major factor driving our choices, but not the only factor.

Often the food log will lead people to big ahas, such as the discovery of patterns they'd never noticed before. One patient, Kristen, never thought of herself as an emotional eater, but became aware of certain triggers related to anxieties about her body. She chose to start seeing a therapist to help her work through a past family history that seemed to have set this pattern in motion.

Another patient, Liam, noticed through his food log that most of his moments of celebration, pleasure, and relaxation were food-driven. He lived in a major city, and most of his entertainment and "self-care" choices were either fine dining or fast food. He already had a therapist, and the three of us worked to help Liam add some new sources of pleasure to his list—for example, he started going on scenic walks in his city and took up tea as a hobby.

The vast majority of us have emotions, both positive and negative, tied up with food. So many of us "eat" our feelings rather than face them. When you change your behavior, all those feelings bubble up into your consciousness. It doesn't always feel great. Over time, your food log can become a space to identify these emotions so that you can work through them, whether on your own, with a friend, or with a professional. (More on this in chapter 7.)

## Habit Foundation 3: Meal Planning

Set a time once a week (for most people it's a weekend day) to sit down with your calendar and plan out all the meals for you and anyone else you'll cook for in the next seven days. Then, get the groceries you'll need or make a plan for shopping.

Meal planning disentangles you from that relentless, never-ending question: *What am I going to eat next?* It allows you to think about your choices once a week, instead of twenty-one times, day in and day out. It allows you make the *majority* of your food choices in an optimal state, when you're well-fed and relaxed. Otherwise, you know what often happens when you get home after a long day of work, open the fridge, and say, "What are we going to eat?" Even if the fridge is full of food, answering that question can be so overwhelming that you either call for takeout, or forget the fresh food and dump a box of spaghetti in a pot.

Your eating habits change surprisingly quickly, with little effort, when what's on your plate is no longer decided based on in-the-moment emotions and hunger.

Remember Gretchen, from chapter 1, who had dieted her way to insulin resistance and debilitating joint pain? She wanted to try weight loss medication as an alternative to diet culture. When I told her the program started with the Habit and Food Foundations, she was really frustrated. Like so many patients, Gretchen's food noise before she started GLP-1s almost *never* shut off—and despite all that chatter, none of it was helping her meet her health goals. She was desperate to free herself, and the Habit Foundations—especially meal planning—at first seemed to be a walk in the wrong direction.

**My Story: The Habits**

*When I first looked at the habits, I thought, "This is just another diet and I'm going to be more food obsessed than ever. Just give me the meds and leave me alone!" But by a month in, I had a completely different perspective.*

**— Gretchen**

"I understand how you feel," I told her. "But this is only our *starting* place." I explained to her that increased focus now would lead to less obsession later. I've never had a patient on this journey who didn't arrive at a place, often very quickly, where they were able to **think less about food than ever before**. Short-term, the medication makes that possible. Long-term, the Habit Foundations make that possible—and with a greater degree of emotional neutrality than ever before.

> ## "Help! I can't plan anything a week in advance!"
>
> Most people I work with quickly adapt to weekly planning, and find it fits comfortably into their lives. But if that's not the season you're in, you can still get a lot of the benefits by using a daily meal planning tool.
>
> You can find one here:
>
>
>
> (You can see what the planner looks like in Appendix B.)

### It's Only Hard at First

If you're thinking, *This sounds like a lot of work*, I hear you. Meal planning requires more time and thought out of the gate than the other two habits. But over time, it gets *so* much easier. Most of us eat the same thing for at least half of our twenty-one meals, week after week. So meal planning is really only labor-intensive when you're making those initial big shifts, figuring out which foods work best for you and your family now. After about three weeks, you'll have set a routine and rhythm, and your planning won't require anything excepts tweaks. Meal planning is *not* meal prep. You don't have everything chopped into perfect little cubes and stacked neatly in containers. The output of meal planning is a grocery shopping list for the week.

Will your planning be perfect? Definitely not. The goal is to follow your plan 80 to 90 percent of the time. Life will require some last-minute changes, and that's fine.

## *Avoid the Most Common Meal Planning Mistake!*

The secret to effective meal planning isn't only selecting options that align with your new way of eating. **It's choosing options that align with your life.**

The planning process starts with a close look at your calendar: Is it a busy week? A stressful one? Which days do you have time to cook? What meals will be eaten out, with less control over choices? Are any food celebrations, like a birthday dinner, on the agenda?

Meal planning is especially helpful for people who are feeding other people. It allows us to come up with meals that satisfy the whole family's needs, instead of falling into the habit of putting together two separate dinners every night. Or worse, defaulting to what your kids want because it's easier.

Gretchen, my patient who was healing from food obsession, was super skeptical about meal planning. She decided to trust me, and leaned into it in a big way in her first weeks. She had her first major payoff three weeks into her injections, when she was still hungry all the time. That week was particularly stressful, and one night she made a last-minute decision to order Shake Shack for her kids. Since she was pretty hungry, at first she thought she'd get a burger for herself, too. But then she remembered she had already defrosted halibut, thanks to her meal plan, and she could probably have it cooked and ready, with a side of green beans, even faster than the food delivery. She also remembered that the following night she'd be having what we call an "off-plan meal" (see chapter 6) at a friend's birthday dinner at one of her favorite restaurants. Because of her planning, the halibut started to sound as good to her as the burger. Was it as fun a meal as Shake Shack? No, but she had planned for it, and she was happy, in the end, to stick to the plan. The experience was really empowering for her, and she felt balance and satisfaction from making a healthy choice that was new to her.

## HOW TO HAVE A NEUTRAL FOOD PLAN

| ✓ THIS: | ✗ NOT THAT: |
|---|---|
| The planner is a helpful tool that allows me to be realistic and diminish stress. | My plan should be ideal and needs to be perfect. |
| It provides a path to accountability. | If I don't think it can be a perfect week, I should avoid planning. |

# CHAPTER 6

# The Food Foundations

## THE FOOD FOUNDATIONS

- Eat protein first.

- Add more vegetables as hunger returns.

- Don't skip meals.

- Don't wait until you're thirsty to drink.

Here's another persistent, unhelpful myth about GLP-1s: *They destroy the pleasure of eating.* Professor Jens Juul Holst, who discovered the GLP-1 hormone, hasn't helped. "What happens is that you lose your appetite and also the pleasure of eating," he told *Wired.* "That may eventually be a problem, that once you've been on this for a year or two, life is so miserably boring that you can't stand it anymore."[1] I've seen this scare quote reprinted many times.

Across hundreds of patients, I have rarely seen this play out beyond the early months of treatment, when nausea and other GI discomfort can contribute to food aversion. For most, hunger and enjoyment of food return, and remain reliable and important parts of daily life. What the drug *does* do is bring hunger back to healthy levels—and, even more importantly, help people heal when the one two punch of diet culture and chronic hunger has led to food obsession.

## There's Nothing Wrong with Eating for Pleasure

Food is delicious and meant to be enjoyed. But it's difficult—maybe even impossible—to maintain a healthy weight when it becomes your *primary* source of pleasure, especially in a world of abundant hyperpalatable food choices. That's why one of the first priorities of the SoWell Method is to help you **rebalance the role of food in your life**. The Food Foundations in this chapter, in combination with GLP-1s, will free you from both restriction and obsession. They will guide you toward choices that support your health and help you feel good while you're adjusting to the medication, and into the future.

The Food Foundations are not rules, they're building blocks: the habits that ground your eating patterns. You won't follow them at every meal for the rest of your life. It's a direction to move in, not zero-sum thinking.

Implementing the Food Foundations *will be so much easier than you ever imagined*. You can build habits readily when your hunger and cravings temporarily fade. This creates the opportunity for a reset, during which you will rediscover (or perhaps discover for the first time in your life) a natural, balanced relationship with food. In chapter 8, we'll complete the rebalancing by helping you add new, nonfood sources of pleasure to your life as well.

Changing your habits still takes preparation and focus—but without all that old neurohormonal chatter distracting you.

## FIND FREEDOM IN FOOD RULES

| ✓ THIS: | ✗ NOT THAT: |
|---|---|
| Food is my fuel. I am eating to live, not living to eat. | Food is my source of joy, comfort, and stress relief. |
| Knowing exactly how to eat helps me to minimize food choice chaos. | Reduced food choices feels like a punishment. |
| Having rules helps me to not act impulsively and to achieve my goal. | Rules are no fun. |

## Food Foundation 1: Eat Your Protein, Ideally First

 **Your Goal:**
20–40 grams of protein at every meal

Protein is important at every step of your GLP-1 journey—in other words, for the rest of your life.

With restrictive dieting, the biggest problem was how to get yourself to *eat less*. In the first three to six months of GLP-1 usage, your biggest problem is how to get yourself to *eat enough*.

This often trips people up, because they're so used to focusing on foods that give them a lot of volume with few calories, aka *volumetrics*. Now, for a brief window, the inverse is true: Calorie density is supportive of your efforts.

Some GLP-1 users lose their appetite or develop aversions to food they used to like. Others have an appetite but get full very quickly. You won't know how your hunger will be affected until you've started the medication, but *everybody* needs to get their protein in. This is a lifetime recommendation.

### Why Protein First?

A study by researchers at Cornell University showed that if you were to take the traditional American meal—a roll followed by a salad, then a meat-based entrée—and flip the order of the courses so you were having the bread last, you would finish the meal with a blood sugar that was lower by about 30 percent. Food order has a dramatic effect on how your body metabolizes a meal, a tool that can help you smooth out those wild swings in blood sugar that force your body to pump out insulin.[2]

---

**WHAT DOES ABOUT 20 GRAMS OF PROTEIN LOOK LIKE?**

2 eggs + 3 egg whites

3 to 4 ounces uncooked meat or salmon

1 cup cooked lentils

1 cup tofu

2 tablespoons protein powder (products vary, so check the label)

¾ cup cottage cheese

7 ounces Greek yogurt

3 packaged mozzarella string cheeses

3 to 4 ounces water-packed tuna

3 ounces (12 medium) cooked shrimp

## Why Protein Is So Important

In the early days, it's about making sure you eat enough to lose weight at a healthy pace and protect your metabolism. But science has revealed protein has broad benefits for both weight loss and maintenance.

**Protein preserves muscle mass.** Any time you lose weight, you lose a mix of muscle and fat. It's not ideal, but that's how the body works. Studies have shown that higher-protein diets preserve muscle mass during energy-deficient states (i.e., weight loss).[3]

**Protein is satiating.** Eating protein leads to a greater release of satiating gut hormones (CCK, PYY, and GLP-1) as compared to eating carbohydrates, and is linked to a proportional increase in fullness and decreased hunger.[4] This isn't so important in your first year on a GLP-1, but in the long term, eating protein first will help you feel full faster and make you less likely to overeat. It also crowds out the carbs, which you want to dial down while healing from metabolic dysfunction.

**Protein promotes weight loss.** Several clinical trials of six to twelve months reported that a high-protein diet provides weight loss effects and can prevent weight regain after weight loss.[5]

---

PATIENT STORY
## Justine, Protein Queen

Justine hated the idea of "protein first." She loved carbs and hated diets, but agreed to pick some high-protein snacks and meals to build into her weekly plan. After a few weeks, she noticed how much better she felt after these meals—and started finding more to add to her diet. Now she's all about her sheet pan eggs with turkey sausage, salmon bowls, high-protein ramen noodles, and protein shakes. She still loves pizza, but now one slice is enough, and she's lost interest in pasta completely. She's been eating like this for a year now, and always enjoys her food.

*How to Pick a Protein Powder*

Protein powders and packaged protein drinks can be a very useful tool, especially in the early days of a GLP-1 journey. Mix them with water or milk, and maybe some berries, and you've got a super-palatable, portable, high-density meal. When my patients don't have much desire to eat, they often find that they can get more excited about a chocolate or blueberry protein shake than a piece of meat or fish. In the long run, is salmon or another whole food a more satisfying choice? Sure, but right now it's most important to get your protein in.

My favorite protein powder for weight loss, maintenance, and muscle-building benefits is **whey protein**. It is a complete protein, derived from milk, and is easily absorbed by the body. In a 2010 study that examined the effects of four protein-based meals on insulin, glucose, appetite, and food intake, whey protein was the clear winner. Four hours after eating one of the four studied proteins (eggs, turkey, tuna, and whey protein) as a liquid meal, the participants were offered a buffet lunch. The whey group ate significantly less than the others.[6] The explanation may lie in the fact that whey proteins have a faster rate of digestion and absorption than other proteins, producing a rapid peak in plasma amino acids, potentially leading to an earlier rise in satiety hormones.

There are two types of whey protein: whey concentrate and whey isolate. I prefer whey isolate because it has a higher protein content and is lower in carbohydrates and nearly lactose-free. It's also the easiest to mix.

There are other protein options:

- **Egg white protein** is an alternative complete protein that is lactose-free. It's very low in fat and carbohydrates, but has a grainy texture that has definitely made it less popular than whey protein.
- **Soy protein**, derived from soybeans, is considered a complete protein. However, studies have shown that whey-based protein supplementation is superior for building muscle.[7]

- **Pea protein** is one of the more popular protein powders, but it is considered an incomplete protein, as it is low in methionine.
- **Collagen protein powder** is also an incomplete protein, lacking in tryptophan. However, it can be beneficial on your weight loss journey, as it has shown improvement in skin elasticity and increased lean body mass.[8]

*Are complete proteins better?*

No, they're just that—complete. Protein is made from twenty building blocks called amino acids. Our body can make eleven of these (known as *nonessential amino acids*), while the other nine (known as *essential amino acids*) have to come from our diet. A food is considered a *complete protein* when it contains all nine essential amino acids. Animal proteins (poultry, fish, beef, eggs, dairy) and soy are complete proteins. Plant-based proteins (from legumes, nuts, seeds, and whole grains) are incomplete.

All that said, you don't have to worry about completing your proteins at each meal. Your goal is a broad mix over the course of the day. When it comes to protein powder, whey may perform the best overall—but palatability and how well you digest a given protein determine what's best for *you*.

---

**TASTY HIGH-PROTEIN SNACK IDEAS**

1. Greek yogurt (add ground flaxseeds for fiber!)
2. Cottage cheese with berries and sliced almonds
3. Deviled eggs
4. Beef or turkey jerky
5. Low-carb tortilla and turkey roll-ups
6. High-protein smoothies—see the recipes in chapter 12!

## Fat and Carbohydrates: The Other Macronutrients

You probably know that protein, fat, and carbohydrates are the three macronutrients in food. For most people on GLP-1 medications, if you get your protein in, you can let **how your body feels** guide your fat and carbohydrate intake.

We used to think fat made us fat and clogged our arteries. We now know that sugar and processed carbs have a much greater negative impact on our health than fat, thanks to research brought to the mainstream by terrific journalists like Gary Taubes, author of *The Case Against Sugar* and many other books on the benefits of low-carb eating, and doctors like endocrinologist Robert Lustig, who wrote *Fat Chance: Beating the Odds Against Sugar, Processed Food, Obesity, and Disease,* among other titles.

To *feel* your best, start slow with fat—not because it's "bad," but because you need to find out how your GLP-1-supported body tolerates it. For some, any kind of fat—even healthy fat—is a trigger for GI issues in the early days. Food logging will help you identify which foods work for you. Don't be afraid that eating fat will get in the way of weight loss—and there's no need to monitor your fat intake, especially if you concentrate on eating the feel-good fats.

---

**FEEL-GOOD FATS**

⊘ **Full-fat dairy products:** Most people tolerate these well, and they provide calorie density in the early days.

⊘ **Wholesome + natural:** Focus on sources such as olive oil, nuts, avocados, and fatty proteins high in omega-3 fatty acids.

NOT-SO-FEEL-GOOD FATS ────────────────

⚠ **Fats + carbs:** Pass on the big plate of fettuccine Alfredo or the hamburger and french fries—these fat-and-carb combos are the most likely to send you running to the bathroom.

⚠ **Processed foods high in inflammatory omega-6 seed oils:** Frequent consumption of high-fat, hyperprocessed junk foods (e.g., cookies, chips, french fries, most mass-produced baked goods) leads to inflammation, insulin resistance, and illness.

### My Story: Too Much of a Good Thing

*I only got diarrhea once. At a Spanish tapas restaurant, I shared multiple dishes of seafood swimming in olive oil and garlic. Even though my portions were small, my system couldn't handle tablespoons of olive oil. I spent the second half of the meal in the bathroom. Not fun.*

— **Jessica, 32, while on her first dose of Wegovy 1.0 mg**

## The Carb Caveat

Most people don't need to fully restrict their carbs. Once you dial up your protein, you can listen to your body for the rest. But there are a couple of caveats to this way of thinking.

## Caveat One: The Quality of Carbs Always Matters

GLP-1 drugs work best, with the most minimal side effects, when your food choices support stable blood sugar levels. The carbs that have the least impact on your blood sugar are those that come from whole foods: vegetables, fruits, legumes, and whole grains. These carbs are bound to fiber, which slows down how quickly they become sugar in your body.

The carbs that spike your blood sugar are highly processed white carbs: sugar, bread, pasta. When you spike your blood sugar while on a GLP-1, the body is easily able to sweep the sugar out of your bloodstream, but it may overcorrect, giving you relative hypoglycemia. When this happens, you may feel hungry, fatigued, nauseated, or lightheaded. If you ate those carbs with a lot of fat, you will feel even worse.

So while most people don't need to count or restrict carbs, you'll always feel your best when you index toward whole foods. And again, get that protein in first so that carbs naturally take second place.

## Caveat Two: Carbs Can Impact Weight Loss

Each person has their own carbohydrate "sweet spot," the amount they can eat that helps them feel their best, enjoy their food, and either lose weight or maintain it. For some people, it's 100 grams total carbs per day; for others, it's 40 grams; for still others, it's 20. My point in sharing these numbers isn't to encourage you to track your carbs, but instead to pay attention to what works for *you*. What works great for one person may not work at all for another.

Many of my GLP-1 patients, especially once they're on their maintenance journey, find a more conscious effort to limit carbs can be supportive. Most never track their macros, but they think about portion control. Some might be fine with vegetables, but find they gain weight if they eat more than one piece of fruit a day. They tinker until they find the sweet spot.

Some of them cut back on carbs as a maintenance tool. For example, my patient Benjamin was a healthy eater whose weight had crept up into the obesity category over the years. At age 35, he couldn't lose no matter what he did. After a year on a semaglutide, he was back in a healthy BMI zone and shifted to maintenance on a low dose. Any time his weight trends upward, he uses a carb counter and limits himself to 40 grams total daily until his weight restabilizes at goal. That's what works for him.

I do have GLP-1 patients who can't lose or lose too slowly unless they consciously restrict carbs. In cases of metabolic dysfunction, such as type 2 diabetes or PCOS, eating low-carb can help speed up the process of healing. As well, for someone with a very sensitive gut, such as those suffering from irritable bowel syndrome (IBS), bloating, or Crohn's disease, low-carb eating can be transformative, fixing years of what the gastroenterologist could not.

If you suffer from any of these issues or are struggling to lose weight after three months and are at risk of giving up, you might give very low-carb eating (less than 20 grams total a day) a try. You can find my guide online here:

---

**TOP WAYS TO FEEL GREAT ON GLP-1s**

( 1 )   Eat your protein first.

( 2 )   Don't drink too much liquid with meals—
         you need that space for nutrition.

( 3 )   Eat regular meals—don't skip breakfast!

( 4 )   Practice mindful eating—notice when you're full and stop.

( 5 )   Watch your intake of fat and carbs, the top culprits
         (along with overeating) for GI distress.

( 6 )   Take a fiber supplement if you have regularity issues.

---

## Food Foundation 2: Add Vegetables and Fruits as Hunger Returns

You have my permission as a doctor to not eat your veggies—at first.

In the long game, you'll welcome back your big salad, your mountain of kale—but when you start a GLP-1, veggie meals and sides may become temporarily off-limits. The medication slows your digestion, and the fiber in vegetables slows it down even more. The result can be nausea and other unpleasant gastric side effects.

Long-term, low-starch veggies will go back to being your primary partners in health, after protein. Fruits will be yours to enjoy. Volumetrics will once again be helpful in keeping you satisfied. But in your first six months, listen to your body. Eat your protein first and add vegetables as you can.

*Can I Eat as Much Fruit and Vegetables as I Feel Like?*

Unlimited fruits and vegetables can pile on a lot of carbs. Young, active people will readily burn them off. But if you're older, or sedentary, even fruits and vegetables can interfere with weight loss, especially if you skimp on the protein.

A friend and colleague of mine is a super-healthy eater. She couldn't understand why she wasn't losing weight. She loved sheet pan meals, and filled her plate with piles of roasted broccoli, onions, and corn, and a few morsels of meat. She'd finish a meal feeling stuffed, only to feel hungry again an hour or two later. I suggested she dial up her protein and dial down the veg. Even though she was eating less food, she ended up being much more satisfied, and able to lose.

And finally, about fruit: It's delicious and a great source of vitamins and some fiber. But with the exception of berries, fruit is full of sugar, so see it for what it is—a quality source of fast carbs, great for after a workout or as a dessert. And like a dessert, it's best eaten at the end of a meal, not at the beginning, to keep your energy and hunger stable.

## Food Foundation 3: Don't Skip Meals

Fasting all day or for part of the day has become a popular and medically respected approach to optimizing health. But on a GLP-1, skipping meals can make you feel terrible. GLP-1s lower your blood sugar—but that means you need to eat at regular intervals to fuel your body. Otherwise, you might start to feel shaky and fatigued, and have difficulty thinking, and you might lose weight too quickly.

But eating constantly won't serve you, either. Follow the two guidelines outlined below to ensure you're keeping your body and blood sugar stable.

*Eat in 12-Hour Windows*

If you have breakfast at 8 a.m., for example, eat lunch and dinner within the next twelve hours, finishing dinner by 8 p.m., and wait twelve hours before eating again. This short fasting window—mostly happening while you sleep—gives your digestive system time to rest. GLP-1s make the downtime extra important, since the meds slow down and initially stress that system.

*More Meals, Fewer Snacks*

Eating three meals a day gives your now-slower digestive system time to do its job. That said, the goal is to feel fueled and satisfied, so follow your instinct on this. If you're approaching hangry and need a snack, eat it.

## Food Foundation 4: Stay Hydrated

It's always good to stay hydrated. But on a GLP-1, you'll need to be more conscious about hydrating yourself than you've been in the past. The same hormonal pathways that regulate hunger regulate thirst, so your body may need water well before you actually feel the urge. Focus on getting 64 ounces a day; this doesn't need to be exclusively from pure water—coffee, tea, and even the occasional diet soda can contribute to your total ounces—but the emphasis should be on water.

You also might find you need electrolytes. If you're drinking enough water (and eating enough) but still feeling fatigued or lightheaded, or you're having muscle cramps, you might not be getting enough salt or other minerals, aka electrolytes. You can buy flavored electrolyte powder to add to water, or simply add a pinch of salt and a citrus twist to a glass of water once a day.

**My Story: Electrolyte Rescue**

*When I got to the highest dose of Wegovy, I started getting foot cramps and cold feet in the 48 hours after injecting. Also fatigue. Taking electrolytes the day of and the day after my injection resolved the issue.*

**— Jason, 43, lost 50 pounds on Zepbound**

## *Speaking of Hydration . . .*
### *Can I Drink Alcohol?*

You can, but you can anticipate that the negative side effects you might have experienced in the past during and after drinking will be worse while on GLP-1s. How *much* worse depends on the individual. You might find that you used to feel great after two glasses of wine, but now can only tolerate one. So start slowly and proceed with caution. You might have less desire to drink as well. The same mechanisms that reduce food cravings on GLP-1s also seem to reduce alcohol cravings. If you do drink, low-sugar beverages—think dry wines and vodka with sugar-free mixers—will help hedge against side effects.

## Celebrations and Off-Plan Meals

Even early in your GLP-1 journey, not every meal will be a mirror reflection of the Food Foundations. There will be special meals, holiday treats, and days when you decide to have the french fries.

I don't call these "cheats." Eating beyond our nutritional needs for pleasure isn't cheating; it's what humans do sometimes, especially when we get together to celebrate. Life is to be lived!

But in your first six months, GLP-1s are only going to let you go so far with recreational eating. If you approach these meals with a free-for-all attitude, you'll likely feel the consequences. So abandon that old diet mindset that tells you, "If you're going to go off-plan, you may as well go all the way."

When eating off-plan, introduce one new element at a time. Instead of having the cocktail, the fried appetizer, the all-carb entrée, and the dessert at your first celebratory meal, **pick one**. It's not about limiting calories, it's about experimenting to see what your gut can handle, which will change over your time on the medication.

What you eat before and after your off-plan meal matters. Don't "save up" and arrive starving—you may end up eating too much, too quickly, and make yourself sick, or might not be able to find anything appetizing on the menu. You won't be able to enjoy yourself if you spend the meal feeling sick or starving, so plan ahead.

If you know you'll be having an off-plan meal, optimize your next meal to help you feel good. (This is what weekly meal planning is for!) For example, you might make egg and cheese bites ahead of time so they're ready for breakfast the morning after. Or if you're having a big, blowout lunch, have easy-to-digest bone broth waiting at home in case you're not hungry enough to eat dinner.

## A Word on Intuitive Eating

Many practitioners promote intuitive eating as a healthy way to heal from diets. This includes fulfilling cravings when you have them, with the idea that over time, foods lose their hold on you when they're not forbidden. These principles have helped many people on their journey to wellness. For people on GLP-1s, though, they can be a bit of a trap.

What happens if you crave cupcakes—but then have no more room in your stomach for nutrition? What happens if you have no appetite at all? There may be times when eating your protein does not feel intuitive—and yet you still need to do it.

Food choice is extremely important in your first six months, to ensure that you get enough nutrition and fuel. You might eat a handful of french fries and find your hunger satisfied, like some of the TikTok influencers I've seen, but that's not healthy eating—it's a potential eating disorder.

That said, three intuitive-eating principles work really well for GLP-1ers.

**1: Be mindful of hunger while you eat.** With each bite, pay close attention to how you feel so that you can stop when you're satisfied. Many of the worst side effects people experience on GLP-1s come from overeating. They've lost the expectation of satiety and are therefore no longer mindful of its signals. Slow down while you eat so that you can "hear" your satiety, and respond to it by putting your fork down. If the meal is delicious, don't waste it—have more later!

**2: Be mindful of how you feel in the hours after eating.** Foods that you've tolerated well in the past, even healthy foods, may not work for you in the early months of taking a GLP-1. Everybody responds differently to the medication.

One patient of mine, after two months on the full dose of Wegovy, was throwing up several times a week, an extreme and unusual reaction. She was convinced she was "allergic to GLP-1s," until we went back and looked at her food log. Every time she ate the famous Jennifer Aniston kale salad—several times a week, because she loved it—she threw up later that day. Her system could no longer tolerate raw kale. Once she stopped eating it, she was fine. This is where your food log can really serve you in the early months, making it easier to spot patterns and switch things up as needed.

**3: As you start to incorporate the Food Foundations into your life, be gentle with yourself.** Life forces you to make a lot of tricky choices every day, and food is sometimes *the least important of all of them*. Keep your perspective, and forget about trying to wake up and "be perfect." The Foundations give you a direction to move in. Don't change everything about how you're eating at once. Maybe it starts with redesigning your breakfast. Then, when that feels comfortable, move on to the next change. Over time, as the medication changes your underlying biology, the behavioral changes will come naturally.

## Your Biology Will Adapt Over Time

How you eat five weeks into your GLP-1 journey isn't how you'll eat five months into your journey, or five years into your journey. Over time, your body will adapt. Your healthy hunger will return, and you'll be able to eat a wider variety of foods without negative side effects. Your underlying health will also improve, and you'll shift focus from losing weight to maintaining your weight, both of which will expand your options.

The Food Foundations are exactly that: a healthy base to build from to suit your individual biology and lifestyle. They're also a safe place to return to if either your labs or the scale start moving in the wrong direction. But in the first year of your journey, stay mindful. Don't panic if at first your diet feels extremely limited. Once you're on a steady dose, rather than continually titrating up, what and how much you can tolerate will expand month by month. Changing the dosage can also help you find the right balance between eating for fuel, eating for pleasure, and eating to lose weight. The whole point of your GLP-1 journey is to improve your quality of life, now and in the future, and enjoying your food is an important part of the equation.

CHAPTER 7

# The Mental Foundations

GLP-1s are powerful medicines, but you know what's even more powerful, and far more complex? The human brain. *Your* brain. When negative thoughts take control, they can lead to behaviors that derail the physical processes that are finally primed to encourage healthy weight loss. You might self-sabotage by overeating or eating foods you know won't set you up for success. You might delay taking your medication, skip doses, skip doctor's appointments, or drop the medication altogether.

The first barrage of negative thoughts often crops up at what I call the **10-Pound Panic**. This is when, 10 pounds down, so many of my patients—both men and women—start to self-sabotage when they're overwhelmed with mental chatter such as:

*This is where it all falls apart every time—I plateau and lose focus!*

*This has been too easy—the drugs will eventually stop working and I'll fail.*

*Why am I doing this when I know I'll gain back the weight??*

*What if I lose access to the medication down the road? What then?*

The red flag announcing we've entered the 10-Pound Panic is often a sudden avoidance of the Habit Foundations. Patients skip weigh-ins, journal less consistently or not at all, or fall short on their weekly meal planning. If you find yourself doing any of these things at the 10-pound mark or beyond, it's time to slow down and ask: *What's going on in my head?*

### My Story: The 10-Pound Panic

*One week I didn't plan my meals and then I really struggled with what to eat. I found myself returning to my old diet mindset, that if I mess up once, it's all over. So I ended up skipping lunch, an old bad habit. I tried to remind myself that the medicine is here to help and that I need to eat normally and not obsess. I do not want to go back to always stressing about food.*

**— Steph, 51, healed joint pain
and insulin resistance**

The 10-Pound Panic is real, and it's reasonable. It results directly from your experiences with diets in the past. Ten pounds is an inflection point, and the end to many weight loss efforts. And regain, as we know, is the rule, not the exception, when it comes to dieting. What I remind my patients of is that they're on a new journey, supported by medicine—and 10 pounds is only the very beginning. It's way too early to be projecting months or years into the future.

But there's a *second* powerful reason these negative thoughts start to bubble up at just the moment when you're seeing success. It's because this is also the moment when *others* start to see your success. Friends and family might give you compliments, or they might share well-meaning concerns. If you share that you're on a GLP-1, they inevitably have lots of questions and an opinion to share.

Managing the mental game doesn't end with the 10-Pound Panic. It's the greatest challenge of weight loss, and for many, it's lifelong. Fortunately, just as obesity medicine offers tools to manage the physical challenges, cognitive behavioral science has developed effective techniques to help us manage the mental game. I'm going to share some of those tools in this chapter, along with other effective strategies my patients have found most helpful for managing the situations and people that trigger them.

## How Thoughts Lead to Actions

Bianca, a 24-year-old patient of mine, never experienced the 10-Pound Panic. She sailed through her weight loss phase in great spirits. She had come to me because her gynecologist knew I'd had success helping patients find relief from PCOS, which was disrupting Bianca's otherwise happy, exciting life working in finance in New York City. Bianca also had significant insulin resistance and was about 40 pounds overweight—and at her young age was already feeling painful inflammation in her joints. We started her on Wegovy and a lower-carb diet. Seven months later, she had lost the weight and reversed both the PCOS and the insulin resistance. The joint pain was gone. We reduced her dose to stop her from losing more weight, and she shifted into maintenance.

Her panic came toward the end of the weight loss phase, when she suddenly began to doubt all the changes she had made. She was worried what she was doing was unhealthy or extreme, despite the fact that she felt great and was eating three meals a day and snacks. Her labs and new BMI of 23 showed optimal health. I asked her to journal her negative thoughts for a week to see if she could pinpoint the trigger—or what cognitive behavioral therapists call "The Event."

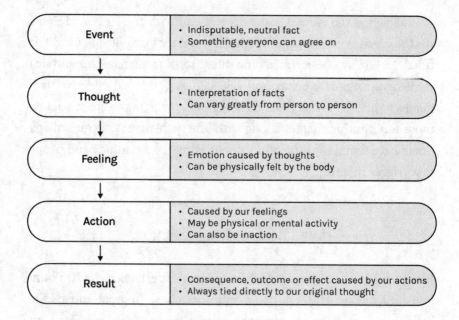

Some event—an activating experience in her life—had led Bianca to . . .

*A thought:* Her new lifestyle was a mistake.

*A feeling:* She felt anxious and heavy in her chest, uncertain.

*An action:* She was skipping weigh-ins and eating snacks she would normally avoid.

*A consequence:* The potential undoing of hard work that had led her to feel physically and mentally better than she ever had.

Bianca soon came to realize that the triggering "event" was her family's reaction to her lifestyle changes. Bianca is Hispanic, and family meals revolved around white rice and tortillas. These were both foods that she had cut way back on, because when she ate a lot of carbs, her joints ached. When her family noticed she was passing on the rice, they were curious at first, and then critical. In particular, her father would not let up on comments about her new weight. "You're wasting away," he kept telling her. She'd go home feeling deflated and rejected by the people she loved most.

*Awareness* is the first step in managing the mental game. The emotional triggers that can send you into a tailspin really aren't always what you might expect. I have patients who tell me they can't wait for the moment that someone first notices and compliments them on their weight loss. Then it happens, and they become insecure and spiral into negative thinking. And that's just one example. Triggers are unique to each individual.

### My Story: Triggers

*One day, about a year into my weight loss, a coworker at the nurses station called me the Incredible Shrinking Woman. I think she meant it as a compliment, but being called out that way at work left me feeling really uneasy. Suddenly I was questioning everything I had done.*

**— Betsy, 125-pound loss**

There's no use in judging yourself for your feelings. You're allowed to have whatever feeling you have. But the goal is to stop the chain reaction of a thought to a feeling to an action to a negative response, or outcome, that doesn't serve us. To do that, you have figure out where the emotions originated, and what actions they're leading to.

That's the path to *managing your triggers* and becoming *intentional in your thinking*.

In Bianca's case, she first had to set some boundaries with her family. She asked her father not to talk to her about her weight. Wary of further critique, she chose not to tell her family that she was using a GLP-1.

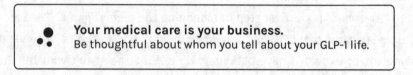

**Your medical care is your business.**
Be thoughtful about whom you tell about your GLP-1 life.

## Two Steps to Rewiring Negative Thoughts

First, write down your negative thoughts as you have them. (For a downloadable worksheet, visit the QR code below.) Do it for a week. I recommend the following prompts, inspired by cognitive behavioral therapy:

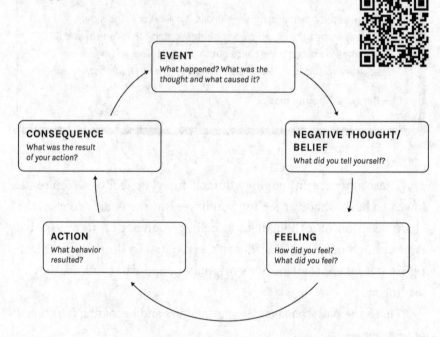

**EVENT**
What happened? What was the thought and what caused it?

**NEGATIVE THOUGHT/ BELIEF**
What did you tell yourself?

**FEELING**
How did you feel? What did you feel?

**ACTION**
What behavior resulted?

**CONSEQUENCE**
What was the result of your action?

Next, **rewire the negative thoughts.** To do this, you need to develop new, healthier scripts to replace your old ones. To help jump-start this process, I asked some of my patients to share the negative thoughts they experienced during their weight loss journeys. Some of the most common are included below, along with some potential alternative scripts. Use them to come up with your own!

## The Top Four Triggers of Negative Thoughts

Here's what my patients tell me are the situations that stir up negative thoughts—and the new scripts they've learned to replace them.

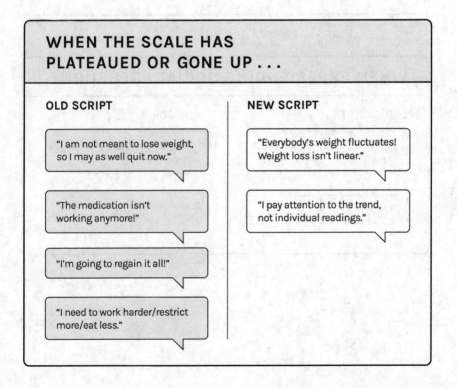

**WHEN THE SCALE HAS PLATEAUED OR GONE UP . . .**

**OLD SCRIPT**

"I am not meant to lose weight, so I may as well quit now."

"The medication isn't working anymore!"

"I'm going to regain it all!"

"I need to work harder/restrict more/eat less."

**NEW SCRIPT**

"Everybody's weight fluctuates! Weight loss isn't linear."

"I pay attention to the trend, not individual readings."

## WHEN MOTIVATION EBBS . . .

**OLD SCRIPT**

"This is taking way too long, when I've put in so much effort. It's not worth it."

"I'm tired of worrying about my health. Live for today!"

**NEW SCRIPT**

"I've been working too hard—I need to give myself a rest or a reward. Besides food, what could it be?"

"Because of the changes I've made, I feel better today and have experienced these benefits: ..."

## WHEN EXPERIENCING SOCIAL PRESSURE . . .

**OLD SCRIPT**

"My family/friends think less of me."

"I'm no fun anymore."

**NEW SCRIPT**

"I'm great company, whatever is on my plate."

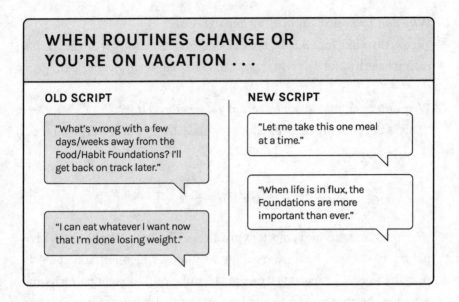

## WHEN ROUTINES CHANGE OR YOU'RE ON VACATION . . .

**OLD SCRIPT**

"What's wrong with a few days/weeks away from the Food/Habit Foundations? I'll get back on track later."

"I can eat whatever I want now that I'm done losing weight."

**NEW SCRIPT**

"Let me take this one meal at a time."

"When life is in flux, the Foundations are more important than ever."

On top of these general negative thoughts, there's a *second* set of negative thoughts that are specific to GLP-1 usage. They're often stirred up by comments from friends or by media headlines. Here are the top four, along with scripts to respond—whether to your own thoughts or the "concerned questions" from others.

*Do you really want to be on a medication for life?*
"Would you say that to someone on a blood pressure medication? Obesity is a disease, and I'm grateful there's finally an effective medicine to treat it—one that is proving to have multiple benefits to my health."

*These drugs are so new. How do you know they are safe?*
"These drugs have been in use for twenty years, with a strong safety record. The scary stories you keep hearing about are in reality extremely rare."

*Why don't you just eat healthy and exercise?*
"Because unlike for GLP-1s, the evidence overwhelmingly suggests that eating healthy and exercising don't lead to long-term weight loss."

*Why don't you just learn to accept your body as it is?*
"This isn't about my size. It's about my underlying health and how I feel."

## Optimize Your Emotional Processing

Negative thoughts and emotions are stressful. That's why so many people try to escape them by reaching for food or alcohol. You can't do that anymore. If you want to rewire old, unhelpful thought patterns and discover the root cause of negative emotions, you have to be willing to spend time with all those uncomfortable thoughts and feelings.

Once again, science provides tools to meet the challenge. Since 1924, neurologists have been able to measure the waves of the brain. What they've learned is that our neurons move at different frequencies, depending on what we're doing. There's an optimal wave speed for changing old thought patterns and generating new insight—and what's even better, with the right activity, we're able to modulate the waves to bring our brains to that state. Neurofeedback machines can literally help people "retrain their brains" and have given us insights into how to get similar results without the machines. For example, if people simply close their eyes and picture something peaceful, in less than half a minute, their brain waves slow down.[1]

There are five distinct speeds of brain waves, but the two that are optimal for integrating new beliefs and patterns are alpha and theta waves. Activities like yoga and deeper meditative states can induce daydream **theta** waves. Your brain produces **alpha** waves when engaged in repetitive activities that operate primarily through muscle memory—activities you barely have to think about to complete, like walking, showering, painting, gardening, needlepoint, doing the dishes, or meditating.

The trouble is, in our busy modern lives, we've outsourced, limited, or abandoned many of these activities. During weight loss, it's important that you find an activity that you enjoy that produces those alpha and theta waves, and schedule time for it daily, or at least weekly. This will give you space to process emotions, reprogram negative thoughts and beliefs, and, maybe most important, relax.

To spark ideas, I often ask people to remember what they loved to do as children. I'll also ask them what their grandparents did to unwind at night. Then I have them build a short list of specific options, so that when they find themselves in "snack mode" or simply feeling antsy, they can reach for it without having to think.

This is critical for managing the mental game, so that by the time you've lost the weight, you've also made some deep changes in how you cope with all the anxieties and obstacles the universe sends your way.

## ACTIVITIES TO GO AHHHH

Make your own list of easy go-tos for relaxation on nights and weekends. Post it on your fridge or somewhere helpful. Everyone's list will be unique, but here are some ideas.

- ⊕ Stretching or exercise
- ⊕ Listening to music
- ⊕ Reading
- ⊕ Self-care (such as baths or skincare)
- ⊕ Showering
- ⊕ Dancing
- ⊕ Hobbies or crafts
  (such as knitting, needlepoint, gardening, or woodworking)

PATIENT STORY
## Fred's LEGOs

Fred mentioned during our appointment that he was struggling not to eat at night as a way to unwind. His life is stressful; he works full-time and lives with his mother, who has dementia. By the time he makes dinner, feeds his mother and puts her to bed, and does the dishes, he just wants to reward himself with snacks in front of the TV. I brought up the idea that he needed to adopt some new hobbies to keep his hands busy and help him relax. I asked him what he loved to do as a kid. His eyes lit up: He loved LEGOs and had recently seen a LEGO kit that had gotten him excited even as an adult. He had thought about buying it, but felt silly. I urged him to try it out as a relaxation technique, and now instead of snacking, he's building.

## One Last Rule to Win the Mental Game

*Be kind to yourself, always.* I hardly ever have patients come to me and say, "Wow, I'm doing great. I'm proud of myself." Instead, they're telling me that they could have worked harder, or done better, or done more.

This isn't a diet you're on. This is the rest of your life. The stumbles are as much a part of the journey as the wins. Note them and move on to the next celebration.

# Your GLP-1 Life

# CHAPTER 8

# A Complete Guide to Feeling Great While Losing Weight on GLP-1s

You've got the prescription. Now what?

Your success with GLP-1s requires so much more knowledge than how to inject the medication, which is often the primary support you get from a med-spa employee or online service, or even from a general practitioner.

What follows is a guide that breaks your first year into phases, with all the info and tips you need to feel great at every step, from your first dose to a celebration of your achievements!

## Prep Phase: The Seven Most Important Things to Do BEFORE You Start the Meds

1. *Record your baseline.* This has two parts. First, **weigh yourself** and record it. Second, ask your doctor or use an at-home testing kit for a **full blood workup** to create a snapshot of your metabolic health prior to starting. At the most basic level, this should include blood glucose (both HbA1c and fasting glucose), cholesterol, and triglycerides. I also like to

include thyroid stimulating hormone, liver enzymes, kidney function, fasting insulin (to help identify insulin resistance), vitamin D, B vitamins, complete blood count (CBC), and iron studies. Finally, consider getting baseline blood pressure and heart rate readings, especially if you are on blood pressure medications.

2. *Get gastrointestinal issues under control.* Don't start a GLP-1 if you're already struggling with reflux, constipation, diarrhea, or gallstones. Resolve these issues first, whether by working with a physician or by making changes to your diet. (Ideally, both!) This is a great time to start **daily fiber supplementation** with a psyllium fiber product. This form of fiber will add bulk to your stool, which helps keep you regular when you're eating less food. The products on the market vary widely in flavor, so now is the time to find one that works for your palate.

3. *Hydrate, hydrate, hydrate.* Dehydration and resulting electrolyte imbalance is one of the most common reasons GLP-1 users experience fatigue in their first months. Because GLP-1s affect your thirst signals, it's easy to forget to drink, **so start building the habit of drinking 64 ounces daily now.** Get yourself a water bottle, an easy visual cue to keep you drinking.

4. *Start working the Habit Foundations.* Daily weigh-ins; food/emotion/hunger logging; weekly meal planning. When you grocery shop after your first weekly meal plan, also **stock up on some of the over-the-counter essentials** to treat the most common GLP-1 side effects (see the first-aid kit recommendations on page 116).

5. ***Start working the Food Foundations.*** Adjust your schedule to accommodate three meals a day, and **stock up on *tasty-to-you* options that will give you 20 to 40 grams of protein** at every meal. If plain, cold chicken breast didn't excite you before you were taking a GLP-1, it's definitely not going to excite you once you are. So think about both protein content and palatability: What will you *enjoy* eating that will also support your well-being?

6. ***Reset your thinking.*** In the Mental Foundations, you learned about rewiring cognitive scripts. It may be too much to start doing that this early in the process. But at this stage, take some time to recognize and honor your past history with weight gain and dieting. Hold space for those feelings, but also remind yourself that you're trying something completely new, with the potential for a completely different experience and outcome. **Trust the science and let the medicine do its work.**

7. ***For women who menstruate: Bulletproof your birth control.*** While this hasn't been studied, anecdotally, surprise pregnancies seem to be an issue on GLP-1s. There are a lot of possible reasons, including the generally positive impact on fertility and the potential disruption to your birth control pill schedule due to GI issues. If you definitely don't want to get pregnant, either **switch to an uninterruptible method**, such as an IUD, or **consider using two forms of birth control**.

## SHOPPING LIST: YOUR GLP-1 FIRST-AID KIT

These are your go-tos for managing symptoms as you titrate up. For any recurrent side effects, stock these at home, but also in your purse or backpack. Refer to the packaging or ask your doctor for proper dosage.

| | |
|---|---|
| **Psyllium fiber** | For gastrointestinal regularity |
| **Sugar-free electrolyte powders or drinks** | For fatigue, dizziness, and muscle cramps often caused by dehydration |
| **Protein powder or premade protein drinks** | For quick, palatable, quality calories when you don't feel like eating, mixed with water, dairy, or milk alternatives, depending on what your stomach handles best |
| **Simethicone pills (e.g., Gas-X)** | For occasional gas |
| **Antacids (e.g., Alka-Seltzer or Tums)** | For reflux and general stomach upset |
| **Bone broth (not stock)** | Electrolytes, collagen, and fat, good for getting a little nutrition in if you're nauseous |
| **Milk of magnesia** | For constipation as needed |
| **Magnesium glycinate** | For daily constipation prevention |

| | |
|---|---|
| Polyethylene glycol (e.g., MiraLAX) | For constipation as needed |
| Loperamide (e.g., Imodium) | For occasional diarrhea |
| Famotidine (e.g., Pepcid) | For fast-acting acid reflux relief; best for occasional reflux |
| Vitamin B6 | For nausea prevention and treatment |
| Papaya enzyme capsules | For sulfur burps (this recommendation is less evidence-based but patients report it helps) |

**Follow this QR code to download a printable shopping list.** ⟶

## What to Know Before You Inject

You are most likely to experience side effects, including fatigue, during the first 48 to 72 hours after injection.

Thursdays and Fridays are the top choices for injection day for many patients, as this allows them to take advantage of the more relaxed weekend schedule to deal with any side effects. And later in the journey, they're happy to have the shot's strongest efficacy over the weekend, when they're most likely to be making spontaneous food choices.

Take the dose any time of day, but be extra careful to get your hydration and protein that day and the next.

Whether you take the drug in the stomach, thigh, or arm will *not* affect your experience on the meds, despite what people may report anecdotally! You'll metabolize the drug the same way at any of the three injection locations. Pick the location that makes it easiest for you to inject.

It doesn't hurt! You'll be injecting into your subcutaneous fat, not your muscle, with a very thin needle. Every so often you might have subtle, transient pain—but I've never had a patient stop because of needle issues, even with patients who've been nervous about injections in the past.

**My Story: Overcoming Needle Nervousness**

I didn't tell Dr. Sowa upfront, but I have a real fear of needles. I had my spouse give me my first shots with the injector because I was so nervous. When I saw how easy it was, I took it over myself.

**—Justin, 40, lost 12 pounds on Zepbound in his first two months**

For specifics on your particular injector pen (or, in the case of compounding pharmacies, the syringe), rely on the package insert and your doctor for guidance.

## Phase I: The Titration Period

You don't start GLP-1s on the full therapeutic dose. If you did, you'd get very sick. Instead, your dose is increased step by step each month—a process called *titration*. For example, Wegovy has five dose steps available, and Zepbound has six. That's because Zepbound's dual agonists are better tolerated by the body, making a higher dose possible. Unlike

Wegovy, Zepbound doesn't have a set therapeutic dose; you start at 2.5 mg and increase until you reach the dose that works best, with 15 mg as the highest available dose. Many clinicians approach Wegovy the same way, but in my experience, most people lose best on the top dose of 2.4 mg.

Some individuals may need to titrate up more slowly; others may not ever need the full dose. The bottom line driving these decisions is that we want the drug to be *efficacious*. Many insurance companies require a second prior authorization at three months; if the patient hasn't lost 5 percent of their total body weight at that point, insurance providers consider the drug ineffective and might deny coverage. In my practice, I prefer to see patients lose 10 percent of their body weight within four months, and we manage titration with that goal in mind.

### For Almost Everybody, the Side Effects Are Manageable!

Titrating up to the full dose as your body adjusts is the hardest part of the GLP-1 journey. But for most patients, a practical self-care program makes this period completely manageable.

Jessie, 32, had already tried GLP-1s once when she came to me. The first time she quit because, in her first weeks on the meds, she experienced terrible diarrhea and stomach pain. When she discussed it with her doctor, the doctor kept telling her she was eating too much. This nonspecific advice left her feeling ashamed, panicked, and helpless.

When she came to me and told me her story, I convinced her to give the meds a second try—with some careful preparation. We reviewed the hunger scale, and she learned to pay close attention to how she was feeling during a meal. We also created a daily protocol of a fiber supplement and a probiotic. Because she travels frequently for work, she put together a complete "go bag" for managing side effects so that she'd be prepared for anything.

When she started on Zepbound, Jessie still experienced diarrhea after her first doses. But this time, she didn't panic. She consulted her food log and saw that high-carbohydrate meals always preceded her worst GI troubles. While titrating up, she avoided fried foods and processed carbohydrates. These changes, along with her consistent morning fiber, got the diarrhea fully under control. Now she's on the full dose of Zepbound, feeling great, and well on her way to a healthy weight.

If Jessie—whose GI issues were among the most extreme I've seen—was able to manage her side effects, I believe almost anyone can.

## Every Experience Is Different

If you experience only mild side effects during titration, yes, the drug is working! You're in the lucky camp of those who tolerate GLP-1s extremely readily.

If you experience moderate to extreme side effects, yes, the drug is working! This is not a sign that you're "allergic" to the medication or that it's incompatible with your body. Side effects, sometimes even very uncomfortable ones, are normal, and you will learn how to manage them. And once you're through the titration period, they're likely to disappear entirely.

## The New Dose Checklist

The first week on a new dose is always the hardest. Your best shot at managing the symptoms is to take some time to plan before your injection.

Think of it as a new self-care routine. In the days before you take a higher dose, pour yourself a cup of tea, sit down with your calendar and your food log, and work through the following list:

**Look forward at your schedule.** What's coming in the week ahead? Get ahead of potential challenges by organizing support or changing your schedule. It's OK to take the dose a day early or a few days late if it helps you avoid potential pitfalls—for example, you may not want your new dose to hit on the busiest or most stressful day of your week.

**Review your food and emotion logs.** Take some time to go deep in your log. If you realize you've been falling behind on your logging, recommit. Have you identified foods or scenarios that trigger side effects?

**Reread the Food Foundations** so that all your best choices are top of mind.

**Plan the week's meals.** You're already doing this every week, but plan meals for new-dose weeks with special care. You may not have much interest in food prep (or eating) during titration, so make sure you've taken that into account by planning easy-to-prepare meals that deliver the protein you need via foods you enjoy.

---

**TOP WAYS TO FEEL GREAT
IN THE 72 HOURS AFTER A NEW DOSE**

You've seen this before, but it's worth repeating!

(1) Eat your protein first.

(2) If you're filling up too quickly, try drinking less liquid during meals and avoiding fizzy drinks.

(3) Eat regular meals—don't skip breakfast!

( 4 )    Practice mindful eating—notice when you're full and stop.

( 5 )    Watch your intake of fat and carbs, the top culprits
        (along with overeating) for GI distress.

( 6 )    Take a fiber supplement if you have gastrointestinal issues.

( 7 )    Take a daily electrolyte supplement.

### The Two-Week Self-Check-In

After two weeks on a new dose, ask yourself if your side effects have resolved enough that you feel comfortable. If not, it may be time to advocate for yourself with your doctor. To streamline their process, many doctors write the prescriptions in advance on a schedule that assumes a new dose each month, with just one refill per dose. But if you're still experiencing moderate to heavy side effects on your current dose, you should wait to move up. Don't be afraid to speak up and ask your doctor if you can slow your titration.

**My Story: Titrate at Your Own Speed**

*I had a trip to Disney planned the same week I was supposed to jump from 1.7 mg to 2.4 mg on Wegovy. I had some pretty significant side effects after the last step up, including fatigue in the 48 hours after the dose, so I asked to stay with the 1.7 mg for another month. There was no reason to rush.*

**—Sara, 46, 25 pounds down and still losing**

Visiting Disney World—or embarking on any other big, activity-intense trip—the same week as a new dose would be hard! But with a

# A GUIDE TO MANAGING THE MOST COMMON SIDE EFFECTS

 ## Nausea

**Daily prevention:** Hydrate with water, sugar-free electrolyte drinks, or bone broth with salt. Consider a daily dose of 15 to 50 mg of vitamin B6. Most nausea can be avoided by limiting carbs and fat, and not eating beyond fullness.

**As-needed treatment:** Occasional Zofran. This is a prescription-strength anti-nausea med you'll need your doctor to prescribe. Use it only for occasional, severe nausea, because it can cause constipation as a side effect.

 ## Diarrhea

**Daily prevention:** Daily psyllium husk, an insoluble fiber, will increase bulk of stools, but you also want a soluble fiber, so look for a supplement that has both. Identify food triggers!

**As-needed treatment:** Hydrate with water and bone broth. Take over-the-counter Imodium (loperamide) as needed; if the maximum daily dose is not improving symptoms, or you're needing to use it more than a few days, talk to your doctor.

 ## Constipation

**Daily prevention:** Take psyllium husk daily and increase water intake. Also consider daily magnesium glycinate at a dose of 100 mg at bedtime (as a bonus, it can help with sleep).

**As-needed treatment:** Milk of magnesia or MiraLAX at bedtime until stools normalize (do not do this longer than one week, unless a doctor tells you to).

 ## Headache

**Daily prevention:** Hydrate with water, sugar-free electrolyte drinks, or bone broth with salt.

**As-needed treatment:** Increase hydration with electrolytes and manage pain with Tylenol or Advil.

 ## Acid reflux

**Daily prevention:** Identify and avoid trigger foods.

**As-needed treatment:** Occasional reflux can be treated with famotidine or antacids, but if reflux is occurring more than three or four times a week, talk to your doctor, who may prescribe taking omeprazole daily for a period of time. Omeprazole is available over the counter (under the brand name Prilosec), but there can be issues with long-term daily use, so it merits a conversation with your doctor.

little planning, you can manage almost anything else in life, even during titration. If fatigue is a side effect for you, schedule naps and quiet time. If nausea is an issue, have electrolytes, vitamin B6, and even Zofran on hand. With each dose, you'll know more about your personal side effect profile and which tricks work best to keep issues in check.

## The Potential Side Effect Your Doctor Is Least Likely to Mention

Three months into her program, my patient Gwen kept journaling about how she felt sad in the afternoons. She told me that in the past, an afternoon snack had always gotten her over this daily emotional hump, but now that wasn't working for her; outside of meals, she didn't have the desire to eat.

Gwen was dealing with something I see in many patients in their first months on a GLP-1: *anhedonia*, or a subtle lack of pleasure. So many people use food as their daily go-to for pleasure, a quick dopamine hit that makes them feel rewarded and relaxed. When Wegovy or Zepbound temporarily reduces the pleasure they get from food, they're left with a void.

### My Story: Emotional Cravings

*When things weren't going well at work, I'd feel a little down and head to the kitchen for an afternoon snack, my old habit for a pick-me-up. But then I'd open the fridge and not find anything appealing. So I'd wander back to my desk in a meh mood, and didn't know what to do about it.*

— Gwen, 38

Once their dosage is established, their favorite foods become palatable again, and the anhedonia fades. And by that time, they've also found some other quick sources of pleasure so they're not reliant on food alone.

## Explore New Sources of Pleasure

Gwen decided to buy a nice teapot and some interesting teas. Now when she hits that afternoon lull, she brews herself a cup and spends a few minutes bird-watching out her back window. I had another patient whose favorite way to relax was to bake cookies. She didn't stop baking entirely, but she moved toward baking gifts for others, and also renewed an old hobby, knitting. Yet another patient joined a paddleball club because he lost his taste for beer, which made spending time at bars a lot less fun.

If you're feeling empty or low because food is less interesting, ask yourself **what other interest you might renew or explore**. A few more ideas:

- Listening to music
- Yoga or meditation
- Drawing, coloring, or painting
- Walking outside or sitting in the sunshine
- Tarot card reading
- Joining a club, such as a book club or mah-jongg group

## Emotional Processing Time

If food has been a coping mechanism, you might also need to address the underlying emotions that come up during this period. (See chapter 7 for activities that support emotional processing.) Logging and journaling can be especially helpful in helping us bring to the surface and wrangle with negative emotions. This habit alone allows most of my patients to grow and learn during titration and beyond. If you find that's not enough, consider seeking out a friend or professional to talk through any negative emotions.

## Phase II: The Steady Dose

After the titration period concludes in four to six months, side effects fade away for most people. This a good thing—and yet it can cause real panic.

"It stopped working!" a patient might tell me when we meet for a six-month check-in. "I'm never nauseated anymore, and this week I've been hungry every single day!"

The distress can be significant. People lose their sense of control, and old cognitive scripts surface: "It's impossible for me to maintain a healthy weight," or "I know I'm the only person the medication won't work for."

I take as much time as needed to reassure them with the facts: Nausea is a *side effect*. Yes, it deters eating, but keeping you feeling nauseated is not the way the GLP-1s are intended to work long-term. Once nausea fades, the agonists continue to do their work, messaging satiety to the brain. They're still slowing digestion, keeping food in the stomach longer so that you feel full longer. The hunger that returns is healthy and normal. People who are genetically predisposed to being thin still have hunger—hunger that is satiated by eating a meal.

"Are you still full after eating?" I ask them. Inevitably, the answer is yes. The medication is working. The trend in their weight is still downward.

*Grab Your Guardrail—The Foundations*

When *you* reach this part of the journey, learn from my patients and try not to panic. This is your new normal. If you do panic, use the Habit and Food Foundations to steady yourself. What you're experiencing are healthy hunger signals. Hopefully you've been working on the Food Foundations since day one, but if not, now is the time to lean in.

Same with the Habit Foundations. Use your food journal to get to know your new patterns, especially with regard to hunger, and look for any emotional issues or lingering side effects that may be keeping you from eating well and consistently.

DANIEL'S STORY
## When Extreme Side Effects Linger

For some patients, side effects linger even after titration—but they decide that living with those side effects is worth it for the health benefits they're getting from the medication. Daniel, a talented writer, decided to try medical weight management after experiencing a major health scare, a pulmonary embolism. "It left me feeling an urgent need to take better care of my health," he said. At 53, he was suffering from sleep apnea and hypertension, and after examining his labs, I diagnosed him with prediabetes and metabolic syndrome. He had a BMI of 37 at 270 pounds.

He started on Wegovy and boosted his protein and vegetable intake. With each dose, he experienced intermittent diarrhea, but it would pass. Then, after two months on the full dose of Wegovy, the diarrhea came roaring back. None of the usual fixes seemed to help him. A colonoscopy confirmed his colon health, suggesting his system was just extremely sensitive to the medication. We dropped him down to a lower dose, which immediately resolved the issue.

Later, when he hit a plateau, we decided to try the higher dose again—but encountered the same problem. At that point we had the conversation:

Did the efficacy at the higher dose outweigh the inconvenience of the occasional diarrhea? He decided it did, and kept losing for a few months on the 2.4 mg dose of Wegovy. Later, when Zepbound was approved by the FDA, he switched over—and his side effects immediately resolved.

Daniel ultimately lost 70 pounds, ending up with a BMI of 28. His glucose levels are back to normal, and the sleep apnea and hypertension are gone.

## Get Your Six-Month Labs—and Celebrate!

Remember how you got those baseline labs? At six months, or after about 40 pounds of weight loss (whichever comes first), run those labs again.

You should see improvement in all the biomarkers of metabolic syndrome and inflammation—with the possible exception of your cholesterol. Sometimes LDL will actually go up after weight loss because of the release of fats into the bloodstream. Don't panic! Continue eating with the Food Foundations as your guidelines, and test again in three to six months.

The best feeling I have as a doctor is delivering the news that liver enzyme, blood sugar, and cholesterol numbers have all normalized. Putting type 2 diabetes into remission. Reversing metabolic syndrome. It's my "why" for being in the field of obesity medicine.

Retest for any abnormalities seen on initial labs to make sure supplementation or treatment has been successful.

## Common Emotional Stumbling Blocks

The GLP-1 journey is both physical and psychological. Following are some of the most common stumbling blocks patients face in their first year.

## COMMON EMOTIONAL
## STUMBLING BLOCKS

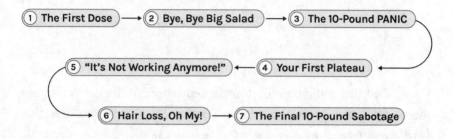

### The First Dose

Many people fill their prescription and get scared, both because of their past experiences with weight loss and because they're trying something new. To set yourself up for success, acknowledge your fears, but make a commitment to educating yourself about this new method and then following through. If needles scare you, ask a loved one to give you your injection.

### Bye-Bye, Big Salad

Suddenly, the big salad or huge plate of greens you equated with "healthy" or "clean" eating in the past now doesn't seem appealing or leads to GI distress. For weeks you may eat mostly protein, perhaps at times (or often) in a processed, artificially sweetened form like a shake because it's what your stomach will tolerate, or you develop a temporary aversion to meat. Sometimes patients struggle with the feeling that they're eating *less* healthfully than they used to. Remind yourself that this is temporary. What's most important in these early months is that you don't let your calories drop so low that you're losing weight too rapidly. Just for this one short period of life, don't worry about "eating your vegetables." Eat protein, supplement with fiber, eat cooked or smaller portions of veggies, and look forward to adding more bulky vegetables back in as soon as you're able—for most, by around six months.

### The 10-Pound Panic

I described this common milestone in depth back in chapter 7: the moment when, after losing about 10 pounds, people often panic. First, this is where things have fallen apart for them in the past. And second, this is when other people start to notice their weight loss, make comments, and ask questions. Self-consciousness combined with past history opens the floodgates to negative thinking. They start forecasting failure in the future, which leads to sabotage in the present. If this happens to you, slow down and breathe. You are very early in the process. It's too soon to know what the future looks like.

### Your First Plateau

At some point a few months in, weight loss inevitably slows and may temporarily stop. You may even register a gain. This is normal. No weight loss process is linear. Continue working the Foundations. Do not stop weighing in. The trend will move back in the right direction—and this plateau almost certainly won't be your last.

### "It's Not Working Anymore!"

Somewhere between the third month of titration up to a year after being on a steady dose, you start to get hungry again; you might anticipate your next meal and experience some food noise. This does not mean the medication has stopped working. Welcome back your hunger while continuing to follow the Food Foundations. Your metabolism is in healthy working order, and you'll continue to lose or maintain.

### Hair Loss, Oh My!

GLP-1s do not cause hair loss—but losing weight does. The scientific term for this is *telogen effluvium*. It's the same phenomena that causes hair loss after childbirth, in which a stressful event (stressful in the sense that it uses lots of your body's resources) triggers hair to move from the growth (anagen) phase into the "resting" (telogen) phase and subsequently sheds. My patients usually notice this around a 40-pound loss, or three to four months into their GLP-1 journey. It can last for up to six months, but the hair generally grows back on its own. Nutritional deficiencies, including too-low protein intake, can worsen the hair loss. In general, the hair cycle will return to normal within six months.

### The Final 10-Pound Sabotage

At about a year, give or take a few months, most people are close to their most important goal—a total loss of 15 to 20 percent of their total body weight. Their health metrics are improved, and they feel terrific. They are approaching the point where they won't lose more weight without making more lifestyle changes. Sometimes we stop here—but often people will have a goal weight in mind that they haven't yet reached. At this point, they start to sabotage themselves with old dieting mindsets. They tell themselves, *I'll be better tomorrow, so that I can lose 5/10/15 more pounds.* If trying to lose more brings up old negative mindsets, or leaves you feeling like normal healthy eating isn't enough or that you need to "try harder," it's time to stop.

## How Do I Know When I'm Done?

After about a year on a steady dose, most of you will stop losing. For some, this is the natural point to end the weight loss phase and shift to planning for lifelong, sustainable maintenance. We'll talk about what that looks like in chapter 12.

For many others, "How do I know when I'm done?" is a more difficult question to answer.

My patient Margaret, 26, was extremely disappointed when she plateaued after a year with a BMI of 28. From a medical point of view, she had made an incredible transformation. She had started her journey with significant obesity, and one year later was at a weight that no longer posed a health risk, confirmed by labs that showed peak metabolic health. But she was worried about what she called her "pooch," saying that it made her dating life uncomfortable.

It was time for Margaret to transition from a weight loss journey to a new journey to confront her weight-related insecurities. I referred her to a therapist who has helped her develop a healthy self-esteem at her current weight.

My patient Andrew represents another extreme. He was a big guy who had steadily gained weight after high school, but who had no issues with his size. He lifted weights and felt healthy at a muscular 225 pounds, but during the pandemic he became sedentary and gained 70 pounds. At his next annual checkup, his blood work suggested nonalcoholic fatty liver syndrome. He was only twenty-nine, but his liver enzymes were double and triple the normal range. Untreated, the condition could eventually progress to cirrhosis, the same liver disease that can result from alcoholism.

When Andrew had lost about 50 pounds on Wegovy, his weight plateaued. He told me he was OK with it; he felt great and was ready to maintain. But when we ran his labs, his enzymes, though improved, were still elevated. He also still had a high-risk BMI.

Given these underlying signals, I encouraged him to work through a food issue that had persisted throughout his program. Andrew was a person who self-soothed and relieved stress by stuffing himself. Since childhood, he could remember feeling calmed by the feeling of being too full. Several times a week, he was ordering takeout and eating well beyond satiety.

I was concerned that, down the road, this behavior could lead to regain and send his labs back in the wrong direction. He agreed to cut back on the fast food and to work on eating slowly and stopping at "satisfied," not "stuffed."

Over time, with great support from his girlfriend—who loved him at every size but wanted him to be healthy—he started to recognize and enjoy moderation. These changes led to more weight loss. Andrew finished his weight loss journey with a BMI of 30— technically still considered overweight, but he maintained a lot of muscle mass from a regular lifting program at the gym, and his labs showed a complete reversal of his fatty liver.

When a patient's weight stabilizes at a BMI that's considered overweight but their labs reflect peak health, I encourage them to shift to maintenance. At this point, focusing on homeostasis—maintaining their new, lower weight for the rest of their lives—will serve their health more than trying to knock off a few more pounds, especially if it sends them down a path of dieting and disordered eating.

Sometimes their other doctors persist in making comments or recommendations about their weight. I prepare them with a script: "Working with an obesity specialist, we agreed that this is a metabolically healthy weight for me."

## A Final Success Factor: Curiosity

I can promise you this: Your GLP-1 journey will be unlike any other weight loss program you've experienced in the past. Pay attention to how you're thinking and feeling along the way—and log or journal as much as you can. That extra level of self-awareness, and the tangible data history it creates, will help you meet changes and challenges with curiosity rather than fear. Your ultimate goal is to finish your weight loss journey with not just a lower number on the scale but a healthy new lifestyle—your new normal.

# CHAPTER 9

# Getting a Prescription and Getting It Covered

I hope that within the next five years, this chapter will no longer be needed because the administrative process of getting and filling a prescription for a GLP-1 medication has become as straightforward as getting a statin for high cholesterol. But for now, getting access to GLP-1s remains difficult. In the United States, insurance coverage limitations, the high cost of the drug, doctor bias, and medication shortages are among the roadblocks to treatment. Getting a prescription will require knowledge and self-advocacy. This chapter will provide you with the tools, but you'll need to bring the persistence.

## Three Questions to Ask Your Insurance Company

Start by calling your insurance company to find out what medication coverage you have. Ask your insurance company the following questions:

**"Do I have anti-obesity medication (AOM) coverage or weight loss medication coverage?"** Ask using both terms— "anti-obesity medication" *and* "weight loss medication"—because the formal terminology varies among insurance companies. If the answer is that yes, you're covered, ask what medications are on your insurance formulary for weight loss medication. (Commonly prescribed medications are Zepbound, Wegovy, Saxenda, Contrave, and Qsymia.)

**"Do I have coverage of Ozempic or Mounjaro?"** Then ask the follow-up: "Do I have to have a diagnosis of type 2 diabetes for the medication to be approved?" Some insurance has historically covered these drugs with a diagnosis of prediabetes or insulin resistance, although that's been less the case since demand for the drugs has surged.

**"What is my deductible? Do I have to meet my deductible before having medication coverage?"** If you're covered, this will help you figure out your potential out-of-pocket cost for the drug.

Whatever you learn from this conversation, don't stop here! Moving through the healthcare system to a diagnosis and prescription can take time, and access to these drugs is expanding rapidly. For example, Medicare—which used to have a blanket ban on weight loss medication coverage—now covers the medication for those patients who have both obesity and cardiovascular disease.

If you're on a company health plan, you can also begin to lobby your human resources department to cover these drugs in the future.

## Finding the Right Doctor

To get and stay on GLP-1s, you need to find the right doctor—one who understands that GLP-1 medications combined with lifestyle changes are often the best, most sustainable way to reverse obesity and unlock the health benefits of losing excess weight. You also want someone whose practice fits your lifestyle and your budget, so that you can maintain the relationship long-term.

Just as important, you need a doctor who is willing and able to fight for your coverage with the insurance company. There are many doctors who would like to prescribe these medications, but don't have the bandwidth to jump through the administrative hoops to get patients covered. This makes your choice of doctor particularly important—and also your commitment to persistent follow-up with them. The squeaky wheel gets the oil.

If you have a primary care physician who is knowledgeable about GLP-1 usage, you're set. But otherwise, working with a doctor who is certified by the American Board of Obesity Medicine (ABOM) ensures that your clinician will be prepared to help you address the unique challenges associated with medical weight management. You can use the ABOM website (https://www.abom.org/) to find an obesity medicine physician near you. Right now, only a tiny percentage of doctors are obesity medicine specialists, but the field is growing rapidly.

### My Story: A Questionable Recommendation

*I have been chronically overweight or obese my entire adulthood and had tried and failed to lose weight for several years after I turned 50. Finally I asked my doctor about GLP-1s, and he said, "I don't like to prescribe those meds because I can't get patients off them." He asked me to try again to lose for six months before he would refer me to an obesity medicine specialist. When I finally visited the specialist almost a year later, since I had to wait for an appointment, she told me that these medications were intended for lifetime use, and that my chronic obesity and family history of type 2 diabetes made me an ideal candidate. I wish I had gotten a second opinion*

*from a better-informed doctor instead of delaying my weight loss*
*for more than a year.*

— **Jonathan, start weight 270 pounds,**
**down 35 pounds after four months on Wegovy**

## Pre-Appointment Checklist

Once you think you've identified the right medical team, there are a few things you'll want to make sure you do before booking your appointment. Many medical offices have detailed information on their websites, but if you can't easily find the answers to the questions below, call the office before you book.

**Identify the qualifications of your medical care team.** Will your appointment be with a doctor, or with a registered nurse or physician's assistant or another professional in the practice? Is the clinician you are planning to see accustomed to dealing with issues of weight management? (See page 136 for advice on how to best identify a qualified medical care team.)

**Figure out how far into the future the office is booking appointments.** Consult the front office of your respective care team to get a better understanding of how far in the future appointments are booked—it's not unusual for there to be a significant wait time for consultations.

**Consult online reviews of your care team.** If you don't know someone personally who can recommend the care team you're considering, check for reviews online. There are plenty of websites where you can get a good idea of a clinician's bedside manner, professionalism, and overall approval rating.

**Get a clear idea of the anticipated finances.** Is the clinician you are looking to consult covered by your insurance? What are the upfront costs of care? Make sure you understand the costs associated with every step, including the initial consultation and any subsequent treatment.

**Document your relevant medical history to bring to your appointment.** This should include your lifetime weight history and any past issues that might affect your experience on a GLP-1 or contraindicate its use. In particular, make sure to mention:

- If you have either of the primary contraindications for GLP-1s: a personal or family history of medullary thyroid cancer or multiple endocrine neoplasia, type 2 (MEN 2)
- Any past or current GI issues (e.g., IBS, pancreatitis, gastroparesis, diverticulitis, constipation, acid reflux)
- If you've had your gallbladder removed
- Past trouble with gallstones or pain after eating
- If you have a weak stomach and/or are prone to nausea or motion sickness

**Document your weight loss history.** Often for both diagnostic and insurance purposes, your doctor will need a detailed history of your prior attempts to lose weight, including information about what program or diet was followed (e.g., WeightWatchers or another weight loss program, specific exercise programs or gym memberships, a low-carb diet, calorie restriction), start and end dates, and your weight before and after the program. Make a comprehensive list and bring it with you to the appointment. A list of programs might look like this:

Name of weight loss programs: Starting date–end date (starting weight, ending weight)

Specific gym/exercise programs/gym memberships: Starting date–end date (starting weight, ending weight)

Counting macros/low-carb diet: Starting date–end date (starting weight, ending weight)

But I also like patients to provide me with a more holistic overview of their weight history, which might look something like this:

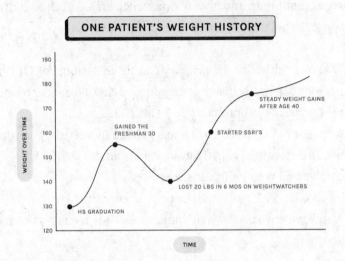

**ONE PATIENT'S WEIGHT HISTORY**

During your appointment, make sure to ask about the titration and prescription process with your doctor:

- Will they write the prescriptions for each titration dose up front, or will you check in each month to make a decision on whether to continue or increase your dose?
- What's the best way to correspond when it comes to prior authorizations and refills?

## Getting Prior Authorization

You're probably familiar with the normal process of getting a prescription filled. Your doctor writes you a script, their office calls it into your pharmacy of choice, and your pharmacy calls you when the medication is available so that you can pick it up.

The process is rarely so simple with GLP-1 medications! Instead, progress often breaks down when the script reaches the pharmacy. They contact your insurance company and are told the drug isn't covered or that it requires prior authorization. Many patients drop out of the process here, assuming this means they have to pay out of pocket for these medications, which cost upward of $1,000 a month.

Typically, insurance plans that cover GLP-1 drugs for weight loss require doctors to submit a request for prior authorization (PA). This is how these for-profit companies limit access to the most expensive drugs. In practice, it creates a huge administrative burden for doctors prescribing these medications, and often leads to eligible patients never getting their prescription filled.

Your doctor's office will initiate and complete the prior authorization request, but you may need to bring this to their attention and follow up. If progress stalls, I recommend making a follow-up appointment to work through the PA together.

In addition, most insurance companies require physicians to include supporting chart notes and documentation with the request.

To submit a prior authorization, physicians can either call insurance companies directly or submit a request for prior authorization on third-party sites like www.CoverMyMeds.health. Depending on the insurance company, it can take as little as a few minutes or up to seven days to hear the outcome of the prior authorization.

## At the Pharmacy

Pharmacists sometimes resent these drugs because they are often difficult to source through distributors. They also carry the bureaucratic headaches of prior authorization and shortages. Be nice to your pharmacist.

The following tips will help you get your script filled promptly.

After your doctor sends in your prescription, confirm your pharmacy has received it, that they have your up-to-date insurance information on file, and that they have the medication in stock. Find out whether you need prior authorization. It's best to give your pharmacy a call or visit them in person. Pharmacy apps do not always display up-to-date and/or correct information about availability.

If your preferred pharmacy doesn't have your medication in stock, try others in your area. I often find that pharmacies located in grocery stores have the best supply.

If you need to switch pharmacies, you don't need your doctor to transfer the prescription for you. Have the new pharmacy call the pharmacy where your doctor originally sent the prescription and request the transfer.

If you're struggling to find your medication, call your local chain pharmacy and ask them to check all of the pharmacies in their database within a 20-mile radius to see if any of those stores have your medication in stock.

---

## PHARMACY PITFALLS TO AVOID WHILE TITRATING UP

⊙ Confirm the dosage you are filling, every time. With multiple prescriptions in the system, pharmacists can get confused.

⊙ Some insurance plans require prior authorization for each titration dose – make sure your doctor is on top of it.

⊙ Don't wait until the last minute; two weeks before it's time for your next refill, call your doctor and your pharmacy to make sure everything is in order.

## When Insurance Companies Deny Coverage After You've Started

Once you've received a prescription, you may need your doctor's help to keep it. Watch for two issues:

- Many companies will require proof of efficacy at three months. Your doctor will need to show that you have lost 5 percent of your total body weight for your insurance coverage to continue.

- Once you reach a healthy BMI, some insurance companies seek to deny coverage because they don't understand that lifetime usage is indicated to maintain your new weight. (You may also encounter doctors who try to take you off the medication because you're "at goal.") Coverage decisions (and prior authorization requests) should be based on your *baseline* BMI, before you started taking a GLP-1. If you are denied continuance of coverage on the basis of your new BMI, your doctor may have to call the insurance company to advocate on your behalf.

## The Trouble with Compounding Pharmacies

Because Wegovy and Mounjaro are expensive and often in shortage, many patients and their clinicians have turned to compounding pharmacies. These pharmacies exist to produce custom formulations of drugs—for example, they might replace a particular ingredient in a drug if a patient has an allergy. However, when a drug is on the FDA shortage list, as GLP-1s were in 2023 and 2024, compounding pharmacists are also allowed to produce drugs that the agency calls "essentially copies."[1] This provision has allowed compounding pharmacies to offer replicas of GLP-1s, despite protests from the originating companies.

Even reputable compounding pharmacies have received warnings from the FDA. Many are producing GLP-1s by combining semaglutide sodium salts instead of the semaglutide base used in the FDA-approved name-brand formulations. These pharmacists point out that combining the salts creates the base and is therefore "essentially a copy" and legal. However, the FDA, along with drug makers Eli Lilly and Novo Nordisk, have warned pharmacies and customers against this practice, saying that these salts have not been through trials and therefore have uncertain safety and efficacy.

If you do work with an online pharmacy, medical spa, or doctor who obtains their GLP-1s from a compounding pharmacy, at least make sure the pharmacy is a **503A state-licensed or 503B FDA-licensed sterile compounding facility**, and that they can provide your doctor with a certificate of analysis for the compounded medication.

Hopefully, GLP-1 drug makers will soon resolve the issues that have driven patients to compounding pharmacies. In late 2024, Eli Lilly took a major step toward easing shortages by making Zepbound available in single-dose vials. (The injector pens, not the drug itself, create the supply constraint.)

From my point of view as a doctor, the controversy over compounding may be distracting us from an even more critical and widespread safety issue: the hazards of working with a clinician who does not evaluate your health holistically before prescribing these medications. Medical spas, which specialize in cosmetic treatments, and online clinicians designed specifically to sell GLP-1 medications often do not have the medical expertise or processes in place to identify whether you're truly a good candidate for the drug and support you in resolving any health issues along the way if you are. As well, they may not offer the support needed to teach you how to inject yourself safely with the proper dose. Be sure you are informed, and stay safe out there, friends.

# CHAPTER 10

# Why Hard Cardio Can Hurt— and What to Do Instead

GLP-1-supported weight loss requires a huge shift in how we think about exercise.

The old thinking went like this: Exercise intensely during your diet to burn enough calories to help achieve your daily 500-calorie deficit. With traditional dieting, getting that deficit wasn't easy, so when it came to exercise, people focused on what burned the most calories— cardio. An hour of hard cardio daily seemed like a good way to balance the ledger without starving yourself.

Enter GLP-1s: Your challenge in the early days is to eat *enough* that you don't lose weight too quickly. Adding a bunch of exercise can actually undermine you. You might get weak or fatigued, or feel nauseated. Sometimes I even recommend that patients cut back their exercise, especially if they've been on a schedule of relentless, grueling cardio. In fact, I make this recommendation whether they're on GLP-1s or not— because we now know that "balancing the ledger" with exercise has never made a significant impact on weight loss.[1] A more holistic understanding of exercise and its impact has additionally revealed that the old thinking doesn't serve our long-term health goals, either.

There's a more effective path than grinding out cardio to protect our metabolism, maintain weight loss long-term, and feel our best. Read on!

## The Revealing Math of Energy Expenditure

The easiest way to understand why our old way of thinking was so limited is to look at the math behind daily energy expenditure.

Total energy expenditure =

Basal metabolic rate (BMR)

+

Thermogenic effect of food

+

Non-exercise activity thermogenesis (NEAT)

+

Exercise

Your **basal metabolic rate (BMR)** is the calories you burn daily to keep your body alive. It comprises the majority (about 60 percent) of the calories you burn in a day.

The **thermogenic effect of food** is what you burn in digestion, about 10 to 15 percent of total daily burn.

**Non-exercise activity thermogenesis (NEAT)** represents the calories you burn from any movement you make as you go about the business of life. On average, it's about 15 percent of your daily burn.[2]

Adding **exercise**—the kind of movement where you intentionally work your heart or your muscles—may contribute another 10 to 30 percent of daily burn.

What that means is that no matter how hard you work out, exercise is always going to be a minor player in total calorie burn. That's the math.

## More Levers, Better Results

Today, instead of concentrating only on exercise as the means to increase daily calorie burn, we've realized we need to look at the whole picture. What other levers can we pull that might be more sustainable and impactful than scheduling big blocks of cardio?

The SoWell Method recommends patients adopt a more active lifestyle in three stages.

## Stage 1: Move More

Early in your GLP-1 program, begin by increasing your NEAT movement.

NEAT is all the calories you burn simply by living your life. It includes everything from fidgeting at your desk to cooking dinner to getting down on the carpet to play with kids to climbing steps. For sedentary individuals, NEAT accounts for about 15 percent of daily burn; however, it can range widely. There can be a difference of up to 2,000 calories a day between two individuals of similar size.[3]

Biology determines some of that difference. If you've ever met someone who "just can't be still," constantly fidgeting, toe-tapping, or pacing, that person will have a higher NEAT. All those tiny motions throughout the day add up. But your occupation makes the biggest difference. Anyone who spends six to eight hours a day in constant motion burns far more calories than those of us who sit at desks most of the day.

Most of us can't change our jobs, but there are many ways we can increase our NEAT expenditure.

## *Walk More*

One easy, already popular route is increasing your daily steps. Use your phone or a step counter to establish your baseline, then look at your day for opportunities to get more steps in. The idea isn't to find an hour when you can take a hike, but instead to fit more activity into life's daily business.

---

**INCREASE YOUR STEPS**
CAN YOU:

⊕ Get off the bus or train one stop early?

⊕ Park at the far end of the lot?

⊕ Take the stairs instead of the elevator or escalator?

⊕ Walk to do errands instead of driving or having items delivered?

⊕ Skip the drive-through and go inside?

⊕ Take 5- to 10-minute walks after meals?

⊕ Walk to a colleague's desk instead of calling or messaging them?

---

None of these take much time or effort on their own, but their cumulative effect can both benefit your daily burn and improve your energy levels. Try to get to 10,000 steps as your daily target. Remember, you don't have to get there right away.

## *Now Add Intensity!*

Next, see where you can add intensity to life's activities.

**MORE WAYS TO INCREASE NEAT**
CAN YOU:

- Increase your walking or stair-climbing speed?
- Carry your groceries instead of using a cart?
- Wear a weighted backpack while walking?
- Move more while sitting at your desk?
- Dance your way through kitchen cleanup?
- Take your kids to the playground instead of playing at home?

You get the picture. Find ways to make everyday life more physically challenging than it was in the past.

## Stage 2: Maintain and Build Muscle

Since the majority of our daily burn is from BMR, it would be ideal if we could increase that number, right?

Three-quarters of the individual variability in BMR can be predicted by lean body mass. That's because muscle burns more calories than fat. So, to maintain or improve our BMR, we need to maintain or grow new muscle. But when individuals with obesity successfully lose weight, their muscle mass usually decreases as their body fat decreases.[4] You can't just lose body fat alone. You also lose lean body mass purely as a function of aging, unless you take steps to prevent muscle loss. What this means is that the long-term trend in BMR for sedentary individuals, but especially those losing weight, is downward.

The good news: Though height, sex, and age are the primary determinants of lean body mass, anyone—of any age or sex—can increase lean muscle mass through weight training to achieve a small bump in BMR. Every 10 pounds of muscle contributes about 60 calories to BMR.[5] Weight training (also known as resistance training) is also the key to preserving muscle while losing weight.

For folks over 55 who are losing weight, it's important to protect muscle to avoid sarcopenia and sarcopenic obesity, which is the condition of having a lot of excess fat and very low muscle mass. This low muscle-to-fat ratio is worse than obesity alone, with an increased risk of adverse health consequences, including cardiovascular metabolic diseases and death from any cause.[6]

## When and How to Start Weight Training

The answer is different for everyone, but in short, you should start when you feel good enough, and are physically and mentally ready to add something new. For many of my patients, weight training as a form of exercise is new territory. It helps to get started *after* they've adjusted to the meds and their new way of eating. Check in with your doctor for the green light on any new activity program.

As a rule of thumb, **don't wait more than six months after you start taking a GLP-1 to start weight training.** If you have any resistance to working with weights, an arbitrary deadline like this can help. If you have previous injuries or current aches, or have not been active in years and feel deconditioned or overwhelmed at the thought of exercise and strength training, consider seeking an evaluation from a physical therapist. In many states, patients no longer need a prescription to establish care.

Other tips to get started:

**Start with simple bodyweight exercises that target the major muscle groups.** There are a plethora of apps and online routines that can support you in this. I love the *New York Times*'s Scientific 7-Minute Workout,[7] a high-intensity workout based on a series of twelve exercises published in a sports medicine journal. Though it was published in 2013, it still hits, and the *Times* has since developed a gentle standing-only version of the exercises, a 9-minute strength version, and an advanced version.

The *Times* routine includes the following widely known body-weight exercises (formerly referred to as calisthenics): jumping jacks, wall sits, push-ups, abdominal crunches, chair steps, squats, tricep chair dips, planks, high knees, lunges, push-ups with rotation, and side planks. While it's true that you can get through all those exercises in 7 minutes, the original authors recommended doing the workout two or three times in a row for the best impact. Still, even one time through may be a challenging starting place, depending on your level of fitness.

**If you want to try a paid app,** look for one like Aaptiv or Apple Fitness that has video demonstrations, interchangeable short and long workouts, and options for both body-weight exercises and dumbbell-assisted workouts.

**Get a gym membership.** This doesn't need to be permanent, but having access to a full weight set can help you figure out what weights and equipment will be crucial to continuing your workouts at home. See if you can find a gym, such as F45, that offers guided weight-lifting classes.

**Get at-home fitness equipment with a subscription that includes weight-training classes, such as Peloton, Mirror, or Tonal.** These are not budget options. They all require an up-front equipment investment and you'll pay monthly fees. But what you get in return is challenging, adaptive, trainer-led workouts in the comfort and convenience of your own home. For many (including me, in fact), that's what it takes to maintain a consistent program.

**Book a few sessions with a personal trainer.** If you can afford it, this is the easiest way to establish a workable program and learn proper form. Some personal trainers do body composition measurement so that you can identify your baseline and a goal to work toward. Physical therapists are a great source of referrals for quality trainers, and so is word of mouth.

**Schedule your training.** Put it in your calendar like any other task. Accountability helps.

**Pay attention to your changing food and hydration needs!** Hydrate (with electrolytes) and plan meals accordingly to avoid the hungries, and eat a good protein-focused meal with some carbs for recovery.

## How to Preserve and Build Muscle Mass

You may have heard that you need to lift heavy weights if you want to *build* muscle. This is not true! The key to building muscle is **lifting to the point of fatigue.**[8] In other words, doing reps until you can't do one more. If you're new to weights, you want to start small, with 2- to 3-pound weights, resistance bands, or body-weight exercises such as push-ups and squats. (The apps and *New York Times* routines recommended on page 151 can provide more detailed guidance.) This will protect you while you develop strength and learn proper form. Aim for two to three resistance-training sessions per week, either weight lifting or body-weight resistance training. But even a single session is better than none!

Studies show that combining resistance training with a high-protein diet is the best way to maintain muscle while losing weight. I recommend 20 to 40 grams of protein per meal (adding up to an overall 70 to 120 grams per day) for most GLP-1 users. When you start regular weight training, aim to eat at the top of that range, or higher. Numerous studies have shown that higher-protein diets protect muscle mass. And in one study of healthy young men restricting calories while on a resistance-based fitness program, the group that ate 1.5 times the Recommended Daily Allowance (RDA) of protein maintained their muscle mass, while the group eating triple the RDA actually gained muscle while losing fat.[9] For reference, the US RDA for sedentary individuals is .36 grams of protein per pound of body weight, or about 60 grams of protein per day for a person weighing 160 pounds.

Rate of weight loss matters when it comes to protecting muscle. Faster isn't better: Aim to lose no more than 1 to 2 percent of your body weight per week. And while weight training might become your focus, cardio continues to matter, for cardiovascular health. Look to break a sweat for at least 20 minutes twice a week—and pay attention to how you feel. Plenty of people love their cardio, and that's great, so long as you enjoy it and it doesn't stop you from resistance training.

*Menopause, Weight Gain, and Muscle*

I work with many female patients who have maintained a healthy weight their entire adult lives, but find themselves gaining 20 pounds or more while their muscle tone declines as they approach and enter menopause. No amount of dieting seems to take off the weight. Though research so far has produced mixed results on whether hormonal changes contribute to this weight gain, menopause symptoms such as sleep deprivation, brain fog, and fatigue can all significantly shift how much someone eats and moves, and how they carry their weight.

Many women who had given up hope see amazing improvements in their body composition when they combine GLP-1s with resistance training. Whenever I work with someone heading into their menopause years, I encourage them to start resistance training right away, so that they've already built the supportive habits before they are fully menopausal. For this group, lifting heavy weights is recommended because it not only builds muscle but protects bone density, which decreases when estrogen levels decline.

Tracy became my patient in her late forties, during perimenopause. When she came to me, she was six months into CrossFit training. She was incredibly strong. However, she also had insulin resistance and about 50 pounds of excess weight. When she started Wegovy, she began losing weight. Eventually she left CrossFit, taking what she had learned about proper form into home workouts using a fitness app. She's now 53, with a lean, muscular build and 20 percent body fat. She hadn't had her period for a year, making her officially menopausal, but she hasn't gained any weight. Her symptoms have been minimal, which she attributes in part to hormone replacement therapy (HRT) and in part to her consistent training program.

---

PATIENT STORY
## From Marathons to Heavy Weights

Halle, age 48 and petite, was a marathon runner, but it had never helped her lose weight, even with careful attention to her macros. Because she had survived breast cancer, her doctor recommended working toward a healthy BMI to ward off recurrence. I prescribed Wegovy, which she started while she was on a break from marathon training. During those initial few months, she shifted to shorter runs, yoga, and some occasional light weights, continuing to exercise throughout her weight loss.

As she increased dosage over the months, Halle sailed smoothly to her goal weight, achieving a total loss of 30 pounds in less than a year. She still loved marathoning, so she had resumed long runs once she was beyond the titration period. I suggested she add heavy weights to her routine, since she was nearing menopause. To get started, she had a DEXA body composition scan and learned that 32 percent of her body mass was fat—at the high end of healthy for her age. She started working with a trainer three times a week. After eight weeks, she got a second scan and learned that she was now at 28 percent fat mass, at the same weight; the difference was new muscle. Today she feels stronger and more capable than ever. And her racing times have improved!

## Do GLP-1s Lead to More Muscle Loss Than Other Weight Loss Methods?

Clickbait news articles, as well as some respected health influencers, have warned GLP-1 dieters that they will lose muscle mass. The truth is that *all weight loss* results in the loss of both muscle and fat.

But do GLP-1 medications result in *more* muscle loss than traditional diets? The science isn't yet conclusive, but the picture that's shaping up should not scare potential users away. It is true that in studies from the two major trials of semaglutide, the percentage of muscle lost among the subgroup who got DEXA scans was slightly higher than seen in "normal" diets—39 to 40 percent of total loss, on average, compared to anywhere from 30 to 40 percent from dieting alone.[10]

But even in those studies, the ratio of lean to fat body mass—in other words, **overall body composition**—improved slightly. Still other studies of semaglutide have shown less muscle loss, and data from the major tirzepatide trial showed that roughly a quarter of the participants' weight loss was muscle, a great outcome compared to any diet.[11]

In summary: The science isn't raising any GLP-1-specific alarms here. *Everyone,* particularly those over age 50, should take steps to maintain muscle mass while losing weight.

## The Magic Number for Maintenance

You've heard many recommendations for how much exercise is needed for optimal health. The Centers for Disease Control and Prevention (CDC) recommend 150 minutes of moderate-intensity exercise a week, including two strength-training sessions. But here's what we know that's specific to people seeking to maintain a weight loss: Members of the National Weight Control Registry who have successfully maintained their loss report engaging in **approximately 60 minutes of exercise a day.**[12]

You're not alone if your reaction to that number is: *That's a lot!* It's triple the CDC's recommendation, and no doubt reflects the fact that chronic dieters have lowered their BMRs. It's reasonable to hope that GLP-1s, combined with a fitness program that emphasizes muscle gain, might lead to differing requirements for this next generation of successful losers.

That said, the data has an undeniable takeaway: **Maintaining a healthy weight requires a vigilant commitment to a healthy lifestyle.** Working your way toward 60 minutes of daily activity *is* attainable, particularly when that number is understood as a combination of NEAT (see page 146) and dedicated exercise time.

We also now know that to be effective, exercise doesn't need to be in a single session. A meta-analysis found that intermittent exercise throughout the day has the same health benefits as continuous activity in terms of fitness, blood pressure, lipids, insulin, and glucose. There is even some evidence that favorable changes in body mass can be attributed to accumulated exercise (small amounts throughout the day).[13]

Just by taking a brisk 10-minute walk after each meal, you'd be halfway to a daily 60 minutes. Walking after meals has also consistently been shown to moderate blood sugar levels.[14] Remember our chapter 1 discussion on the relationship between insulin, glucose, and fat storage? It appears that post-meal movement is the most effective way to help insulin grab up glucose and use it for energy, instead of letting it linger in the blood and lead to fat storage.

## Measuring Your Progress

Just as you kicked off your weight loss program by recording a starting weight and getting labs, it is helpful to get a baseline body composition analysis—a measurement of what percentage of your body is fat mass, muscle mass, and sometimes bone mass—before you start weight training. The ability to track whether you're building muscle in such a concrete way can encourage you to persist over time, and provides important data about whether your program is working to improve your ratio of muscle to fat.

Back in chapter 4, we talked about moving away from an "ideal" BMI as a goal. The same holds true for body composition: It's more about where you started and where you are going. I track my patients' body composition to make sure they are preserving muscle mass during weight loss. As they get closer to their goal weight, or we start asking "When should you stop losing?," body fat composition can help guide us and assist us in setting new goals.

While there's no set standard in medicine for ideal fat percentage, the Obesity Medicine Association has established the following classifications:[15]

|  | Women | Men |
|---|---|---|
| Athlete | 15 to 19% | 10 to 14% |
| Fitness | 20 to 24% | 15 to 19% |
| Acceptable | 25 to 29% | 20 to 24% |
| Pre-obesity | 30 to 34% | 25 to 29% |
| Obesity | >35% | >30% |

The most accurate, accessible method to measure body composition these days is a **DEXA scan** (DEXA stands for dual X-ray absorptiometry),[16] a quick test that requires zero prep. A scan costs anywhere from $200 to $300 at commercial testing locations that you can find by googling or asking your doctor. (Insurance may cover a DEXA scan if you're over 50 and at high risk for a bone issue like osteoporosis. Again, ask your doctor.) You lie down as an X-ray scans you, and you get a report that includes your fat mass, your fat-free tissue mass, and your bone mineral content.

Next best is an in-office or in-gym **bioelectrical impedance analysis** (BIA), which measures body composition (fat mass versus lean mass) using a low-level electrical current that changes voltage as it encounters different types of tissue. Brands like InBody and Seca offer a multicompartment analysis (aka 4C model) that calculates fat mass, lean body mass, and hydration status. Gyms and other commercial providers charge anywhere from $49 to $99 to administer these tests.

**Skinfold analysis**, also known as a caliper test, isn't as accurate as the tests above but costs less and is offered by many gyms and personal trainers. The practitioner uses calipers to measure subcutaneous fat at several sites on the body. Because skin fat is proportional to total body fat, those measurements can be used to calculate your overall body composition. The trouble is that accuracy decreases as BMI increases. (Also, not everybody enjoys the experience of having a stranger pinch and measure their inches of fat.) Similarly, **waist circumference testing** is convenient and inexpensive, but may not be accurate. Still, either test can help you track change over time, particularly if you stick with the same practitioner.

**At-home body-fat scales** can measure your total body fat along with your weight. The user experience is identical to that with a standard scale: You step on the scale and read the display (some brands deliver the information in an app). But how accurate are they?

A 2023 study tested fourteen at-home body-fat scales and concluded that "All body fat scales, even the top-ranked devices, demonstrated enough error that you should still be cautious when interpreting the results of an individual test, as well as changes detected by the scale over time."[17] However, the authors also suggested that these scales could be helpful if used in conjunction with other metrics, including body weight, waist circumference, exercise performance, and mood. You can't beat the method for convenience and cost, especially if you're in the market for a new scale anyway. The top-performing scales in the study were the Omron HBF-516, Tanita BC-568 InnerScan, and Tanita UM-081.

And finally, there's the easiest metric of all: **Pay attention to how your clothes are fitting.** If they're getting looser while the scale stays the same, you're increasing your muscle mass and your body composition is improving.

## Start Small, Bring Friends

Many people have emotional baggage when it comes to exercise, a product of those same weight-related fears and insecurities that make the SoWell Habit Foundations a huge revelation for so many. If you're not ready to invest in weights, head to a gym, or see your body composition rendered in black-and-white on a printout, don't let that stop you from getting started.

Your first goal is so simple: *Move more.* Those first steps can be as small as you need them to be: a walk after dinner, a single push-up on your knees, ten biceps curls with a soup can as a weight. Just get started. When you feel ready for more, asking a friend or family member to join you is a great way to face down the fear, have fun, and be accountable for taking better care of yourself, now and long into the future.

# CHAPTER 11

# Maintaining for Life

After a year using the SoWell Method with GLP-1s, you can expect a few common outcomes. You will have lost 10 to 20 percent (or more) of your total body weight. You will be meaningfully healthier, measured by labs and by how you feel. And finally: You will have questions. In particular, about how to ensure that you never have to lose the weight again. This chapter is designed to set you up for success long term.

## What to Do When You Stop Losing

In about 12 to 18 months, the natural weight loss brought about by your personal combination of lifestyle changes and GLP-1 medication will come to a halt. You will plateau. At this point, it's time to answer a few questions.

### Am I at a healthy weight?

Weight health can only be defined by you, in conversation with your doctor. When I have a patient who has stopped losing, and who has already lost 15 percent of their body weight, with labs indicating metabolic health and remission of any weight-related illness, I counsel them to consider shifting to maintenance—no matter what their BMI is, or whether they're wearing the size clothing they had hoped to. Your weight loss journey ends when your health goals have been met, and another journey continues from there: the journey of self-acceptance, which might still include new goals around building strength and physical fitness.

**For maintenance, should my dosage change?**
There are a number of different strategies for the long term. The FDA has approved these drugs for lifelong usage. Trial data shows you need to stay on the drug to maintain, and the majority of people will do best on the full, FDA-approved dose. That said, there are outliers.

In my practice, I help some patients titrate down until they find the dose that allows them to comfortably maintain. There are a few reasons to do this: It helps manage costs for those who are paying out of pocket. Some patients still experience mild side effects, and they feel better on a lower dose. In some cases, particularly with tirzepatide, patients *need* to lower their dose to stop themselves from losing. For everybody, there's some comfort in knowing that if you ever experience regain or find efficacy diminishes, you can titrate up again.

A small subset of my patients—about 10 percent—are able to come off GLP-1s completely. What these patients generally have in common is a very active lifestyle, one that incorporates strength training. Also in this category are people who were not chronically overweight since childhood, but who gained weight after a medical event, such as childbirth or an injury, or because they needed a medication that had weight gain as a side effect. Even among this group, we monitor their weight over time and treat regain by going back on their medication.

The challenge of titrating down is that—until we have studies around maintenance dosing strategies—it requires you to have a practitioner who can work closely with you, over time, to troubleshoot the dosing individually. They may also need to wrangle with your insurance company, some of which require maintenance on the full dose to maintain coverage. For those working with a general practitioner or a specialist with a traditional high-volume practice, you might not get the level of attention that makes this fine-tuning possible. Staying on a consistent dose might be your best bet.

The other challenge in backing off the therapeutic dose for maintenance is that there's no science yet about what works best. With study, we might learn that an every-10-day dosing strategy works better than a similar amount once a week, or any number of other best practices. But for now, we just don't know. Slow experimentation is the only way to figure out what works best for an individual patient. Further studies will come, but slowly, since there's little incentive for the companies who make these drugs to fund them.

### Do I have more weight to lose?

You've got some options. If you have been using liraglutide or semaglutide, you can ask your clinician about switching to tirzepatide, which allows you to move to a higher dose. This often jump-starts a new phase of weight loss. As well, even more effective medications in this class are in the FDA-approval pipeline.

Review the Habit and Food Foundations. A simple return to daily food logging and weekly meal planning is often enough to move into a second phase of losing. Review your logs to see whether there are comfortable changes you can make to bring your eating more in line with the Foundations, more of the time.

Finally, consider your overall activity level. You can add more movement or increase the intensity of your current activities—with the caution that any change you make should be moderate and sustainable over time. Exercising to the point of injury or burnout is not going to serve you long term.

### Have I adopted an active lifestyle?

Weight health almost always requires physical activity. It's really hard to be sedentary and be healthy, particularly as we age. Even on GLP-1s, fitness plays an essential role in maintaining your new weight and aging well. If you haven't already put the framework offered in chapter 10 into action, get to it.

**Have I identified other weight-related issues that I need to address?** Reducing the physical compulsion to eat often reveals the powerful emotional impulses at work in our relationship with food. Likewise, your changing body might stir up unexpected feelings, fears, and desires. If you've found that to be the case, consider working with a therapist to talk through the emotional side of the journey forward.

## Navigating the Unknown

Most of my patients maintain their loss with ease, especially compared to their previous experiences. They've had a year to rewire their brain, and make new habits and foundations routine, plus they're still supported by their GLP-1. They feel great and settle comfortably into a new lifestyle that works for them. They keep weighing daily, and there's not a lot of surprise on the scale.

And then . . . somewhere between six months and a year into their stable weight, something happens. Life delivers one of those guaranteed-to-come "life events," and they're suddenly navigating the unknown. The event could be positive (a promotion at work, a change of address) or negative (the loss of a loved one, a medical issue), but either way, it brings the stress of rapid change. These are the periods of instability in which regain is most likely to happen—yes, even while on GLP-1s.

You can't stop change from happening—but you can **learn to identify the red flags** that suggest your maintenance is at risk, so that you can take steps and, if needed, ask for help.

## Watch for Red Flags

My patient Beth had lost 75 pounds during a two-year period, and maintained that loss with ease for another two years. She came to see me once a quarter, always with a track record of daily weigh-ins.

Then one quarter, she showed up for a visit and told me she had stopped weighing herself two months ago.

### Red Flag 1: You Skip Daily Weigh-Ins

Beth, who was in her early forties, explained that she'd had two big life changes since we'd last met. Weeks after starting a new job, she had also switched to a new birth control pill, her doctor's recommendation to manage worsening premenstrual issues. She had been stressed about the change, because her doctor warned that the new pill was likely to cause weight gain, but she knew she needed to prioritize her mental health.

On the new pill, she rapidly gained 8 pounds. At that point she told herself that it was "reasonable" to stop weighing in; she already had enough stress and didn't want the number to upset her further. She started trying to gauge her weight by how her clothes fit, which had led to more stress because her pants felt tight and she thought she had gained even more.

During our appointment, she finally weighed in and learned she hadn't gained weight since the initial jump. This eased her anxiety, which had increased substantially over the weeks. When I gently suggested that ceasing to weigh in was a stress response, rather than a sensible way to manage the impact of a new medication, she agreed. "It seems obvious now, but I needed someone to point it out to me," she said. "The data really does help." It became clear that the new medication had taken away her sense of control, allowing an emotional relationship with the scale to resurface.

Together we decided to increase her dosage temporarily to help her take off the 8 pounds, and she opted for monthly visits until her habits and health were back on track. I also suggested she take our conversation into her weekly therapy appointment.

**Action steps for Red Flag 1:** Professional help is great, if you have it, but there are powerful steps you can take on your own. If you notice yourself skipping daily weigh-ins, use your journal to explore the practical or emotional factors that are holding you back from doing the things that have been proven to work. Revisit the Mental Foundations in chapter 7. And if you've stopped weighing in entirely, talk the problem through with a trusted loved one who can help you get back on track.

### Red Flag 2: You Don't Fill Your Script or Delay Taking Your Shot

My patient Fred came in having regained 10 pounds. He told me he had gotten too busy to get his medication, and that he had "fallen off the wagon." We dug into it a little, and he told me that his wife's mother had died. He had spent six weeks single-parenting his tween daughter while his wife nursed her mother in hospice. To make things more challenging, his wife had been the one who handled the family's prescriptions.

Another patient stopped taking her medication twice, first when she had a stressful period at work, and again when she had a big move. The reasons she listed for stopping were practical—that she hadn't found a pharmacy yet in her new city and that she was too busy with work commitments. But lying beneath those reasons was a history of childhood trauma that made it difficult for her to manage emotional stress.

**Action steps for Red Flag 2:** Sometimes upheaval creates real practical barriers to filling and taking your prescription. Build as much ease into the process as possible: Can you automate regular delivery through the mail, or move your prescription to a pharmacy that's closer or has better hours? Put a reminder in your calendar for a few days ahead of when you need to refill so you have time to plan and can make sure you're not missing a dose.

When the roadblock between you and your medication is emotional, this is the moment to revisit your whys. Bring in trusted friends and advisors. If you haven't had an accountability buddy along the journey, now is the time to find one. As well, make an appointment to discuss the issue with your doctor.

## Red Flag 3: You're Not Eating Well

If you suddenly find yourself overindulging in your favorite comfort food after months of not thinking about it, you know change is in the air.

My patient Mark had maintained a 50-pound weight loss for more than two years, continuing on the full dose of Wegovy, when he rapidly gained 5 pounds. During a period of significant stress at work, coupled with caring for his sick dog, he had stopped using his meal delivery service or doing any grocery shopping. This happens to people a lot, even when they have their meals automated with a service. When our brain gets overwhelmed, even picking from a list of options or reading a meal service's emails feels like too much.

With an empty fridge, Mark started raiding the work snack pantry and picking up deli subs and chips—his comfort foods of choice—on his way home for work. The first time it happened, he noticed and resumed food logging. But three days of logging subs and junk food left him feeling guilty, so he stopped logging and leaned further into poor choices.

During times of grief, heartache, and stress, gains sometimes happen. We want the chaos outside to be mirrored by chaos inside. Accept it, don't judge it. That makes it so much easier to quickly adjust course as the ground beneath you settles. Fortunately, Mark hadn't stopped weighing in, and hitting the 5-pound mark triggered something in him. He decided to return to the Foundations, eating the same few protein-focused meals on repeat for a few weeks so that he didn't need to make choices or think about food much at all.

**Actions steps for Red Flag 3:** Recommit to the Habit and Food Foundations. Pick some favorite healthy recipes and give weekly meal planning extra attention. The more you plan, the less your food choices will be driven by your emotional impulses.

### Red Flag 4: You Want to Skip Your Medication to Go on Vacation or Celebrate a Big Event

If you're thinking that you want to skip your medication for a week or two to better enjoy a blowout vacation or wedding weekend, this is a red flag that often reflects old patterns of restrict-restrict-indulge behavior. What often happens is that a planned "short break" leads to a long break, and weight gain.

**Action step for Red Flag 4:** Rewrite the cognitive script that tells you that overindulgence in food and drink is the only way to enjoy a real vacation. You can enjoy both on vacation—in moderation. Lean into the travel activities that give you the most pleasure, whether that's relaxing with family, exploring a new city, trying new sports, or enjoying your natural environment. If your vacation would be "boring" without a lot of alcohol, rethink the vacation!

To keep yourself anchored in health, pack a travel scale along with your toothbrush—easy-breezy daily habits, remember? When my patients follow this advice, they come home and tell me, "I can't believe it—I had the best time!" and "This is the first time I've come home from vacation actually feeling rested and refreshed!"

> **CHECKLIST:**
> **WHEN SH\*T HITS THE FAN**
>
> When your routines are in chaos and the red flags start flying, you need structure. Lean on the Foundations. To save yourself from overwhelm, follow this checklist daily:
>
> ⊕ Weigh in.
>
> ⊕ Eat 20 to 40 grams of protein per meal.
>
> ⊕ Log food and emotions.
>
> ⊕ Read and repeat your "whys."

## Dealing with Planned or Unplanned Medication Interruptions

If you need a medical procedure involving anesthesia, you should stop taking your GLP-1 medication seven days before your appointment, according to guidance from the American Society of Anesthesiologists.[1] Without this pause, the fear is that the delay in gastric emptying caused by GLP-1s would result in food sitting in the stomach longer than the "fast before midnight" rule accounts for, especially if the shot is taken in the 72 hours leading up to surgery.

Despite this guidance, I've had patients who were told by a doctor to stop their medication up to four weeks prior. This is misinformed and would totally disrupt re-initiation of the medication. If you are told to pause your medication more than one week, ask the physician who prescribed your medication to update your anesthesiology team on current guidance. To achieve the seven-day pause, I recommend that you move up or back your medication by one or two days weekly before your procedure, to limit the disruption as much as possible.

At some point, you may face a longer interruption to your meds. Due to finances, changes in insurance, or shortages, you may lose access to your medication. Women may need to go off their meds for an extended period for pregnancy and breastfeeding. These interruptions can be scary, but you do have options.

**Titrate down.** It's better for the body to come off the medication slowly, and while you titrate down, you can clean up your diet and really focus on strength training to help maintain while you're off the medication. If you have to make an out-of-pocket purchase, talk to your doctor about how to make it last longer.

**Try another weight loss med.** GLP-1s are the best, but they're not the only. Another medication like Qsymia or Contrave, or even a blood sugar stabilizer like metformin, may be able to help you maintain during an interruption. Talk through the options with your doctor.

**Shift to a very-low-carb diet.** While most people won't stick with such a restrictive plan long-term, it's a great option for short-term interruptions, such as pregnancy or an interim loss of insurance coverage. Taking the carbs out of your diet will reduce hunger and keep your blood sugar stable, mirroring the effects of GLP-1s.

# Recipes and Dining Out

CHAPTER 12

# Simple, Easy Meals for When You Don't Feel Like Eating

For the first four to eight months of your GLP-1 life, file away your fancy cookbooks—but don't *throw* them away. If cooking is an important part of your life, your desire to experiment in the kitchen will eventually return. But when it comes to food, this period in your eating life will be all about simplicity. (Again, lean on those Food Foundations for now.)

Here are the four strategies that we use at SoWell to get patients through those months where they don't have much interest in eating, let alone cooking.

## Strategy 1: Pick Three

You aren't going to want to spend much time thinking about eating. So when you do your weekly meal planning, pick three of each kind of meal (breakfast, lunch, and dinner), and put them on repeat until you're sick of them. Then pick three more. You're much more likely to eat when you take all the decision-making out of it.

## Strategy 2: One Thing, Many Ways

Buy or prepare some basic preferred proteins that you can keep in the fridge all week and turn into a number of meals. My personal favorite is shredded chicken—you'll see it in my Buffalo Chicken Salad recipe on page 189, but I also throw it in soups, top salads with it, and roll it into wraps. It's incredibly versatile. Your favorite might be a deli-style creamy salad (think egg salad, tuna salad, or chicken salad), or a big container of meaty tomato sauce that you eat plain topped with ricotta one day and serve alongside a little pasta or potato another. Check out the chart on page 175 for a great list of ideas to put this strategy into action.

## Strategy 3: Comfort Foods, But Make It Protein

When you really don't want to eat, foods that mimic snacks and desserts tend to still hold some appeal—so let's make healthy, high-protein versions. These foods aren't the building blocks for your long-term epicurean life, but right now they're easy to make and can really hit the spot.

Protein powders, Greek yogurt, cottage cheese, and fruit can be blended together to make an unlimited range of protein-packed meals, customized to your taste. Sugar-alternative sweeteners and sugar-free pudding mixes can make it feel even more "comfort," but if you want to avoid the processed stuff, you can simply mix cottage cheese or Greek yogurt with berries, nuts, cinnamon, and a dash of vanilla extract. If you need more protein, add a scoop of protein powder. Puddings become even more delicious with toppings—try sliced almonds, chia seeds, pumpkin seeds, hemp hearts, berries, bananas, and/or unsweetened shredded coconut.

When it comes to dairy products, I always recommend full-fat versions because they are closer to the whole food and provide the most nutrition. But if you prefer the taste of low-fat versions or find they're easier on your stomach, go for it.

## Strategy 4: Bone Broth

If you're fighting nausea or find yourself unable to eat, reach for bone broth. It has 12 grams of protein per cup, so you'll get at least some nutrition and stay hydrated. Just make sure to buy **bone broth**, not regular broth, which has very little nutrition. You can make your own, but it requires a minimum of 12 hours of cooking on the stove. You can speed up the time using a pressure cooker, but I recommend you buy some to have on hand—convenience is important in the early days. Soups are a comforting option at all times, and great for family meals, served with bread and butter on the side for hungry kids.

# NO-COOK PROTEINS
### STORE-BOUGHT AND READY TO ASSEMBLE AND EAT

| YOU HAVE | | YOU COULD MAKE |
| --- | --- | --- |
| Rotisserie chicken | → | Salads, sandwiches, pulled chicken |
| Chicken, tuna, whitefish, and egg salads | → | Grab-and-go lunches as salads, sandwiches, and wraps |
| Pulled pork, pulled chicken, carnitas | → | Salads, tacos, cauliflower rice bowls |
| Cooked shrimp | → | Shrimp cocktail, stir-fry, tacos, scampi |

| YOU HAVE | | YOU COULD MAKE |
|---|---|---|
| Deli turkey, roast beef, ham, cheeses, Italian salami | → | Sandwiches, salads, charcuterie boards |
| Hard-boiled eggs | → | Salads, sandwiches, deviled eggs |
| Egg bites | → | Low-carb egg wraps |
| Baked/seasoned tofu | → | A sheet pan dinner, in a simmer sauce with veggies, stir-fry, salads |
| Feta and goat cheese | → | Add to salads and eggs, turn into a sheet pan dinner with tomatoes, asparagus, and broccoli |
| Cottage cheese | → | Make puddings and creamy dips, add to scrambled eggs |
| Yogurt | → | Plain or with berries |
| Smoked fish | → | Salads, wraps, on seed crackers |
| Sausage and meatballs | → | In tomato sauce with ricotta and mozzarella to make lasagna-like layered dishes |

# SoWell Recipes

All of the recipes included here supply at least 20 grams of protein per serving. They're simple to make and designed to be palatable and readily digestible for people in the early stages of their GLP-1 journey—but they can be enjoyed by anyone, anytime!

## SMOOTHIES

The combinations for protein-packed smoothies are limitless following this equation:

1 cup water, milk, or milk alternative

\+

1 serving protein powder

\+

½ cup Greek yogurt (can also use cottage cheese or silken tofu)

\+

½ cup fresh or frozen fruit (optional)

\+

½ cup fresh or frozen vegetables such as spinach,
zucchini, or cauliflower (optional)

\+

1 cup ice cubes (optional)

\+

1 tablespoon nut butter, chia seeds, or flaxseeds (optional)

\+

½ to 1 teaspoon cinnamon, vanilla, or cocoa powder (optional)

That basic equation will produce a smoothie with approximately 40 to 50 grams of protein, depending on your choice of milk. Following are a few of our favorite flavor combinations. Just combine all of the ingredients in a blender, blend until creamy, pour into a glass, and enjoy!

## PBJ

1 cup water or milk
1 serving vanilla protein powder
½ cup Greek yogurt or
    cottage cheese
½ cup frozen berries
1 cup ice cubes
1 tablespoon peanut putter
1 tablespoon chia seeds

## The Jungle
## (Dragon Fruit + Spinach)

1 cup water or milk
1 serving vanilla protein powder
½ cup Greek yogurt or
    cottage cheese
½ cup frozen dragon fruit
    (pitaya) chunks
½ cup frozen spinach
1 cup ice cubes

## Cinnamon Banana

1 cup water or milk
1 serving vanilla protein powder
½ cup Greek yogurt or
    cottage cheese
1 small banana
1 cup ice cubes
1 tablespoon chia seeds
½ teaspoon cinnamon

## Chocolate Zucchini

1 cup water or milk
1 serving chocolate protein powder
½ cup Greek yogurt or
    cottage cheese
½ cup frozen zucchini
1 cup ice cubes
1 tablespoon chia seeds
1 tablespoon cocoa powder
    (optional, for extra flavor)

## EGGS & BREAKFAST

Eggs and breakfast foods are a powerhouse in the early days of GLP-1 weight loss, providing an easy and palatable protein base. These "breakfasts" can make an excellent meal any time of the day.

### Creamy Cottage Cheese Egg Bites

These may feel reminiscent of a popular coffee chain egg bite, but my friends and family tell me they like it even better! You can customize the recipe below by adding ¼ cup of any of the following toppings before cooking: chopped cooked bacon, sausage, spinach, tomatoes, onions, or bell peppers.

The cooked bites can be stored in an airtight container for up to 5 days and reheated in the microwave.

6 eggs

1 cup cottage cheese (4%)

½ cup shredded cheese of your choice

¼ cup almond flour

Preheat the oven to 300°F. Grease a nonstick muffin pan (I like using avocado oil cooking spray). Bring a kettle of water to boiling, then pour enough water into a 9 x 13-inch baking dish to fill it halfway. Carefully place the dish on the lower rack of the oven. (This will create steam in the oven, helping to make the eggs nice and fluffy.)

In a blender, combine eggs, cottage cheese, shredded cheese, and almond flour. Blend until smooth. Pour the egg mixture evenly into the muffin tin, filling each cup about ¾ full. If adding toppings, sprinkle them on top and use a spoon to help push them down a little bit, so that the egg mixture just covers the toppings.

Place the muffin tin on the middle rack of the oven, baking for 20 to 25 minutes, until eggs are set. Let eggs cool, about 5 minutes, and then carefully remove them from the tin.

Serves 4 (12 muffins total)

## Sausage, Egg, and Spinach Bake

1 pound breakfast sausage

2 cups fresh spinach, chopped

3 Roma tomatoes, chopped

6 green onions, chopped

10 eggs

½ cup shredded cheese of your choice (optional)

½ teaspoon garlic powder

Salt and pepper to taste

Preheat the oven to 350°F, then lightly grease a 13 x 8-inch baking dish. In a skillet over medium heat, brown and crumble the sausage until fully cooked. Add spinach, tomatoes, and onion to the skillet. Combine and cook until the vegetables are soft, about 2 minutes. Pour the meat and vegetable mixture into the baking dish.

In a separate bowl, crack 10 eggs and whisk well. Stir in shredded cheese, if using, then pour the egg mixture over the meat and vegetables in the baking dish.

Place in the oven and bake 25 to 30 minutes, until eggs are fully set.

Serves about 8

## High-Protein Oatmeal

Oatmeal is a tasty, high-fiber meal, and with a serving of protein powder, it becomes even more satiating. Top your bowl with chia seeds, sliced almonds, or berries for additional flavor.

½ cup old-fashioned rolled oats          1 serving vanilla protein powder
1 cup water or milk (any kind)

In a small pot, boil water or milk. Add in oats, reduce heat to medium, and stir occasionally. Once the oats are thick, typically about 5 minutes, remove from heat and stir in protein powder.

Serves 1

## Protein Pancakes

These don't taste exactly like traditional pancakes—they taste even better and won't leave you feeling sluggish and hungry 20 minutes after your meal.

¾ cup almond flour                    1 teaspoon baking powder
½ cup cottage cheese                  1 teaspoon butter or oil
2 large eggs
1 teaspoon vanilla extract

In a blender or food processor, combine the ingredients until smooth. Preheat a skillet or griddle over medium heat. Lightly coat with butter or oil. Pour about ¼ cup of batter onto the skillet per pancake, and cook for 2 to 3 minutes until edges look set. Flip the pancakes and cook for an additional 1 to 2 minutes, or until cooked through.

Serves 2

## PUDDINGS

For both the protein-packed pudding variations below, mix the ingredients in a medium bowl until completely blended, then cover the bowl. Let set in the fridge for 30 minutes before enjoying. *Each recipe makes 1 serving.*

### Vanilla Pudding

½ packet sugar-free vanilla
   pudding mix
1 cup milk of your choice
1 serving vanilla protein powder

Serves 1

### Chocolate Yogurt Pudding

⅔ cup Greek yogurt
1 serving chocolate protein powder

## MEAL PREP PROTEIN STAPLES

### Shredded Chicken

This is my absolute favorite meal-prep protein, because it can be used in so many ways: salads, sandwiches, soups—or for easily upping the protein content of just about any dish. One pound of breasts yields about three cups of shredded chicken.

| 1 pound boneless, skinless chicken breasts | Salt and pepper to taste |
| 2 tablespoons olive oil | 1 to 2 cups of chicken broth or water |

Season the chicken with salt and pepper. Heat the olive oil in a medium skillet on medium heat. Place the chicken in the skillet for 5 minutes, then use tongs to flip the chicken, cooking an additional 5 minutes. Add the chicken broth to the skillet and bring the liquid to a gentle boil. Once boiling, cover the pot and reduce the heat to low.

Cook chicken for an additional 8 to 10 minutes, or until chicken is cooked through. Let the chicken cool slightly and then shred the meat using two forks.

Store in an airtight container in the fridge or freezer.

Serves 4

## Bone Broth

Bone broth can be made with a variety of animal bones, but to keep things simple this recipe relies on beef marrow bones. Feel free to mix it up, focusing on bones that have a lot of cartilage, tissue, and marrow, which will create the protein-rich gelatin that makes bone broth a nutritional superstar. The recipe below is basic, but you can get creative by adding any seasoning you like. I like warming spices such as Chinese five spice and ginger. If you have a pressure cooker, you can speed things up: Cook on high for four hours, then allow for natural pressure release.

| 3 to 5 pounds of beef marrow bones | 3 to 4 stalks celery |
| 1 onion, halved | 8 to 10 cups water (or enough to cover the bones) |
| 1 bulb of garlic, quartered | Salt and pepper to taste |
| 1 carrot, in chunks | |

Preheat the oven to broil, then spread the bones onto a large sheet pan. Broil the bones on your oven's middle rack for about 5 minutes, then flip and return to the oven for 5 more minutes, or until the bones are browned.

Using tongs, move the hot bones to the slow cooker, then add the onion, garlic, carrot, celery, and water. Cook on low for at least 12 or up to 24 hours. (The longer you cook, the richer the broth.) Allow to cool, then strain the broth through a fine mesh strainer into a large pot. Once cool, skim the fat off the top. Freeze broth into ice cube trays, then store in ziplock bags. Whenever you need a snack, you can pull out a few cubes, put in a mug, and pop it in the microwave. If stored in the refrigerator, the broth will keep for three days.

Serves 8 to 10

## Slow-Cooked Pulled Pork

These smoky, tomatoey flavors are reminiscent of traditional pork tinga, minus the potatoes and chorizo. Pork tenderloin cooks relatively quickly and lets you scale up the recipe easily as needed. This pulled pork is delicious in tacos, burritos, salads, and bowls. Serve with your favorite toppings, such as sour cream, shredded cheese, pickled onion, shredded lettuce, pico de gallo, fresh cilantro, and pickled or fresh jalapeños.

2 tablespoons olive oil

1 medium onion

3 to 5 garlic cloves, finely chopped

1 teaspoon table salt

1 teaspoon ground cumin

1 teaspoon dried oregano

½ teaspoon smoked paprika

1 cup tomato puree or chopped tomatoes

1 canned chipotle pepper in adobo sauce, chopped (for less heat, 1 to 2 tablespoons adobo sauce)

2 pounds pork tenderloin (2 tenderloins, each cut in half)

2 bay leaves

In a medium skillet, heat the olive oil over medium heat. Add the onion and garlic, and cook until the onion begins to soften, 3 to 5 minutes. Stir in the salt, cumin, oregano, and paprika, and cook until the spices become fragrant, about 3 minutes more. Stir in the tomato puree and the chipotle.

Transfer the sauce to a slow cooker. Nestle the pork and bay leaves into the mixture. Cover and cook on low until the pork is tender, 3 to 4 hours.

Remove the pork from the sauce and transfer it to a work surface. Use two forks to shred the meat, then return it to the slow cooker and stir it into the sauce. Simmer for 5 to 10 minutes more before serving.

Serves 6 to 8

## SOUPS AND STEWS

### Spicy Lentil Stew

Even people who didn't grow up with lentils quickly adopt them as comfort food. They're soft, savory, filling, and full of protein and fiber.

1 tablespoon olive oil
¼ cup onion, chopped
5 garlic cloves, minced
1 cup celery, chopped
1 tablespoon tomato paste
4 cups stock of your choice (or bone broth for extra protein)

1½ cups dried brown or red lentils
1 teaspoon paprika
½ teaspoon curry powder
¼ teaspoon ground cumin
½ to 1 cup spinach, chopped
Salt and black pepper

In a soup pot, heat the oil over medium heat. Add the onion and cook for 5 minutes. Add the garlic and celery and cook, stirring occasionally, for 10 minutes more. Stir in the tomato paste, then the stock. Add the lentils and increase the heat to high. Bring to a gentle boil, then cover and cook for 20 minutes. Stir in the paprika, curry powder, and cumin. Stir in the spinach, wait 5 minutes, then serve and enjoy!

Serves 6

## Tortilla Soup

My family loves this recipe! Everyone helps themselves to a topping bar with chopped cilantro, cubed avocado, shredded cheese, sour cream or Greek yogurt, and tortilla strips. You can assemble any toppings you like—it's a party in a bowl.

2 tablespoons olive oil

1 yellow or white onion, chopped

3 garlic cloves, chopped

¼ teaspoon cumin

½ teaspoon chili powder

4 cups chicken broth

1 (14-ounce) can diced tomatoes (ideally, fire roasted and with green chiles)

2 cups shredded chicken (see recipe under Meal Prep Protein Staples, above)

1 (16-ounce) can of black beans (optional)

1 cup frozen corn (optional)

Heat the olive oil in a large pot over medium heat. Add the chopped onion and garlic, and cook until softened, about 5 minutes. Stir in the cumin and chili powder, cooking for another 1 to 2 minutes. Stir in diced tomatoes and chicken broth, and bring to a boil.

Reduce heat, cover, and simmer for 30 minutes.

Carefully ladle the hot soup into a blender, and blend until smooth (you may also use an immersion blender directly in the pot).

Pour soup back into the pot, adding black beans, corn, and shredded chicken. Top with desired toppings.

Serves 4

## 20-Minute Chicken Soup

While I love chicken soup from scratch, this version is a tasty, nourishing way to get in protein and veggies, in no time.

2 tablespoons olive oil
1 yellow or white onion, finely diced
3 garlic cloves, minced
2 carrots, peeled and diced
2 celery stalks, diced
6 cups chicken broth (or bone broth for extra protein)

2 cups shredded chicken (see recipe under Meal Prep Protein Staples, above)
2 teaspoons dried parsley
½ teaspoon dried oregano
½ teaspoon dried basil
Salt and pepper to taste
Fresh parsley, chopped (for garnish)

Heat the olive oil in a large pot over medium heat. Add the onion, carrots, and celery, sautéing for about 3 to 5 minutes until the vegetables are softened. Add the garlic and cook for another minute. Stir in the dried parsley, oregano, and basil. Pour in the chicken stock.

Bring the mixture to a boil, then reduce heat to low to simmer. Add in shredded chicken and cook for an additional 15 minutes. Add salt and pepper to taste, and garnish with fresh parsley.

Serves 4

## Lasagna Soup

This fun take on lasagna will please even people who say soup isn't a meal. It's satisfying and shares the flavor profile of the classic dish—but is a lot less likely to leave you with a stomachache.

2 tablespoons unsalted butter
1 medium onion, diced
2 garlic cloves, minced
Sea salt and freshly ground black pepper
1 pound ground beef
4 cups beef stock

2½ cups marinara sauce
½ cup heavy cream
½ cup full-fat ricotta cheese, plus more for serving
½ cup shredded Parmesan cheese
¼ cup chopped fresh basil

In a large pot, melt the butter over medium-low heat. Add the onion, garlic, and a pinch each of salt and pepper. Cook until the onion is translucent, or 5 to 8 minutes. Turn the heat up to medium-high, and add the ground beef. Cook until browned (7 to 10 minutes), breaking up the meat as it cooks. Drain excess grease from the pot.

Add the stock and marinara to the pot and bring to a boil. Stir in the cream and ricotta. Reduce the heat to maintain a simmer and cook for 30 to 45 minutes. Taste and season with salt and pepper. Serve in bowls, topped with the basil, Parmesan cheese, and extra ricotta.

Serves 7

## Ground Turkey Chili

Who doesn't like chili for dinner? Both kids and grownups like to pick their own toppings, so don't be limited by this recipe. Try chopped radish, shredded lettuce, cilantro, pickled jalapeños, or onions. Creativity, personal preference, and what's in your fridge are your best guides.

1 tablespoon olive oil
1 large onion, chopped
1 red bell pepper, sliced
2 garlic cloves, minced
2 pounds ground turkey
1 (28-ounce) can diced tomatoes, including the juice
1½ cups beef stock (or other stock of your choice)
3 tablespoons tomato paste

2 tablespoons taco seasoning
1 teaspoon table salt
¾ teaspoon black pepper
½ teaspoon chili powder
4 ounces cheddar cheese, shredded, for serving
8 ounces sour cream or plain Greek yogurt, for serving
½ cup fresh parsley, chopped, for serving

In a large nonstick pan or skillet, heat the olive oil over medium heat. Add the onion, bell pepper, and garlic, and cook until fragrant, 1 to 2 minutes. Increase the heat to high and add the ground turkey. Cook, breaking up the meat as it cooks, until mostly browned, or about 8 minutes.

Add the tomatoes, stock, tomato paste, taco seasoning, salt, black pepper, and chili powder, and reduce the heat to low. Cover and simmer for 1½ to 2 hours, until thick. Taste and adjust the seasonings.

Ladle into bowls and serve topped with the cheddar cheese, sour cream, and parsley.

Serves 8

## SALADS

I love an easy deli-style egg or chicken salad to help patients get a large amount of protein in a small container. They can be added over lettuce-based salads, served in a low-carb wrap, or, sometimes best, eaten alone.

### Egg Salad

8 hard-boiled eggs, peeled
½ cup mayonnaise
1 tablespoon Dijon mustard

2 tablespoons fresh dill, chopped
Salt and pepper to taste

Chop the hard-boiled eggs and place them in a large bowl. Add mayonnaise, mustard, and dill. Season with salt and pepper to taste.

Serves 2–3

### Honey Mustard Chicken Salad

½ cup Greek yogurt (2% or higher)
¼ cup mayonnaise
1 tablespoon honey
2 tablespoons Dijon mustard

3 cups shredded chicken
2 stalks celery, diced
¼ white onion, minced
Salt and pepper to taste

In a small bowl, mix Greek yogurt, mayonnaise, honey, and Dijon mustard. In a large bowl, mix together the chicken, celery, and onion. Add contents of small bowl to large bowl and stir well. Season with salt and pepper to taste.

Serves 4

## Chef Salad

This classic salad always feels like a treat. If you like, omit the vinegar and oil, and use your dressing of choice.

| | |
|---|---|
| ½ to 1 head romaine lettuce, chopped | 1 large hard-boiled egg, chopped |
| 1 slice bacon, cooked and chopped | Salt and black pepper |
| ½ medium avocado, chopped | 1 tablespoon olive oil |
| 3½ ounces cooked chicken breast, chopped | 1 tablespoon apple cider vinegar |
| 1 ounce cheddar cheese, shredded | |

Place the lettuce in a large salad bowl. Top the lettuce with the bacon, avocado, chicken, cheese, and egg. Season with salt and pepper to taste. Drizzle with the olive oil and vinegar, and enjoy.

Serves 1

## Dr. Sowa's Go-to Chopped Buffalo Chicken Salad

No one is going to call this gourmet, but it has a ton of flavor and keeps me going for hours. I keep precooked grilled chicken strips and a jar of pickled onions in my refrigerator so I always have this as an option for a last-minute meal. I could eat this salad on repeat every day (and some weeks, I do!). The combination of crunch and heat turns boring chopped chicken salad into something that both satisfies and satiates me.

3 to 4 ounces grilled chicken breast, chopped

1 to 3 tablespoons buffalo sauce (to taste)

1 ounce crumbled feta cheese

Pickled onions

1 cup sliced cucumber

½ cup diced tomatoes

In a large bowl, combine the chicken, buffalo sauce, feta, pickled onions, cucumber, and tomatoes.

Serves 1

## Taco Salad

Taco salad is another staple in my household—colorful, palatable, and easy to adapt depending on your hunger level and how much roughage you can handle. As always, feel free to bring in more toppings, such as chopped cilantro, radishes, or corn.

1 pound ground beef

½ (1.25-ounce) packet taco seasoning

¾ cup water

2 cups lettuce, chopped

½ avocado, sliced

2 tablespoons red onion, chopped

½ lime

½ cup grated cheese of your choice

¼ cup sour cream

Heat a large skillet over medium-high heat. Add the ground beef and cook until browned, 7 to 10 minutes. Add the taco seasoning and water, and simmer for 5 minutes, or until most of the water has been absorbed.

Arrange lettuce, avocado, and onion on each serving plate. Top with the meat mixture, cheese, and sour cream, then serve.

Serves 4

## FAMILY DINNER

### Sheet Pan Caprese Chicken Thighs

This riff on the classic tomato-basil-mozzarella combo is as simple and pared down to make as it is impressively tasty to eat. Pesto gets all the credit here. Half the container goes on the sheet pan, and the other half gets tossed with linguine as a side. I've opted for burrata over mozzarella, because I love its creaminess and how easy it is to tear and toss.

1 tablespoon olive oil
12 ounces grape tomatoes
1 (7-ounce) container pesto
Salt and black pepper
8 bone-in, skin-on chicken thighs, patted dry
8 ounces burrata cheese

¼ cup grated Parmesan, Grana Padano, or Pecorino Romano cheese
½ cup fresh basil leaves
8 ounces uncooked linguine (optional)

Preheat the oven to 450°F. Position a rack in the lower third of the oven. Brush a baking sheet with the olive oil.

Place the tomatoes in a medium bowl. Add a tablespoon or two of the pesto and a pinch each of salt and pepper, and gently toss to coat.

Lightly season the chicken thighs with salt and pepper, and place them on the prepared baking sheet. Set aside half the remaining pesto for the pasta (if not using pasta, save the extra for garnish), then rub the rest all over the chicken, including under the skin—lifting it up, pushing a bit of pesto underneath, then smoothing the skin back down. Arrange the chicken skin-side up and roast for 15 minutes.

Remove the baking sheet from the oven and add the tomatoes, scattering them around the chicken. Return the pan to the oven and roast for 15 to 20 minutes more, until the chicken skin is golden and crispy and the meat is cooked through (it should register an internal temperature of 165°F).

Remove the pan from the oven. If there's a lot of liquid in the pan, pour some out by gently tilting the pan. Scatter the burrata over the chicken and tomatoes, sprinkle the cheese on top, and toss the basil leaves all around.

If desired, bring a large pot of water to a boil and cook the pasta according to the package directions. Drain and toss with the reserved pesto.

Serve the pasta alongside the chicken and tomatoes.

Serves 4

## Peanut-Ginger Salmon with Smashed Cucumber Salad

This super-speedy (just 15 minutes in the oven) and easy meal is also a little elegant thanks to the cucumber and avocado salad on the side.

4 salmon fillets, skin on
Olive oil
Salt and black pepper
6 Persian (mini) cucumbers
1 avocado

3 to 4 tablespoons low-sodium soy sauce
1 to 2 tablespoons toasted sesame oil
Juice of 1 lime
Peanut-ginger sauce (recipe follows)
Thinly sliced jalapeño, for serving (optional)

Preheat the oven to 425°F. Line a baking sheet with parchment paper or aluminum foil.

Place the salmon fillets on the prepared baking sheet and brush them with olive oil. Sprinkle each fillet with a pinch each of salt and pepper. Roast until cooked through, typically 7 minutes per ½ inch of thickness (about 15 minutes for a 1-inch-thick fillet).

Meanwhile, gently smash the cucumbers (a rolling pin works well for this), then cut or break them into bite-size pieces and place them in a serving bowl. Cut the avocado into bite-size pieces and add it to the bowl. Add the soy sauce, sesame oil, lime juice, and a pinch of salt, and toss. Taste and adjust the seasoning if necessary.

Drizzle the cooked salmon with the peanut-ginger sauce, scatter jalapeño on top, if desired, and serve with the cucumber-avocado salad alongside.

Serves 4

## Peanut-Ginger Sauce

½ cup no-sugar-added peanut butter
3 tablespoons rice vinegar
3 tablespoons fresh lime juice
2 to 3 tablespoons soy sauce
1 tablespoon toasted sesame oil

1 tablespoon sriracha, or a pinch of red pepper flakes
½ to 1 small garlic clove, grated
1 to 2 teaspoons fresh ginger, grated
¼ teaspoon table salt, plus more as needed
Water or coconut milk (optional)

In a medium bowl, whisk together the peanut butter, vinegar, lime juice, soy sauce, sesame oil, sriracha, garlic, ginger, and salt until smooth. If the sauce seems too thick, thin it with water or coconut milk, if desired. Taste and adjust the seasoning. If not using immediately, transfer the sauce to an airtight container and store in the refrigerator for up to 1 week or in the freezer for up to 2 months. If frozen, thaw overnight in the fridge before using.

Makes about 1 cup

## Mediterranean Stovetop Shrimp or Tofu

Lightning-fast and incredibly tasty, this recipe can easily be doubled for guests or halved when you're dining solo. Keep shrimp in the freezer to make this anytime. To thaw frozen shrimp, place them in a large bowl of cold water and let stand for 5 to 10 minutes, then drain them, refill the bowl with cold water, and let stand for 2 to 3 minutes more. If any remain partially frozen, rinse them under cold water until thawed. Drain, pat dry, and proceed with the recipe. Serve this over cauliflower rice or Palmini brand mashed hearts of palm. Opt for tofu and skip the goat cheese if you're eating vegan.

2 tablespoons olive oil

1 clove garlic, minced

Pinch of red pepper flakes

¼ cup pitted olives, chopped (any type you like)

1 tablespoon capers

12 ounces peeled shrimp, or 12 ounces extra-firm tofu, pressed and cut into cubes or domino-shaped slabs

Salt and black pepper

½ to ¾ cup fresh tomatoes, chopped

¼ cup crumbled goat cheese, for garnish (optional)

Chopped fresh herbs, such as parsley or chives, for garnish (optional)

Cauliflower rice or cooked quinoa, for serving

In a medium skillet, combine the olive oil, garlic, and red pepper flakes. Cook over medium-low heat until the garlic is fragrant, about 1 minute. Add the olives and capers, and cook for 1 minute. Season the shrimp with a pinch each of salt and pepper, and add it to the pan, trying to keep the shrimp in a single layer, if possible. Add the tomatoes and cook for 3 to 4 minutes, then turn the shrimp over and cook until they are pink and cooked through, 3 to 4 minutes.

Transfer to a serving dish and garnish with the goat cheese and herbs, if desired. Serve over cauliflower rice or quinoa.

Serves 2

# CHAPTER 13

# A Guide to Dining Out

The Food Foundations are the key to taking your healthy habits on the road—whether to fine-dining restaurants, casual diners or chain restaurants, airports, or hotels. No matter where you go, you can find options to support protein-first eating—especially if you do a little legwork beforehand. The most important success factor for eating well when you're not at home is *planning*.

## Restaurant Meals

The goal is to be able to open a menu and find something, no matter what kind of restaurant you're in. If your old go-to favorites have been pastas and risotto, consider it an adventure to explore the other side of the menu where mains like grilled fish, pork chops, steak, and roasted chicken live. If you don't see any mains that'll work, try revisiting the starters and first courses—when you don't have much appetite, you'll find they make a great meal. And if your food comes with starchy sides, you should absolutely have a taste—but as usual, protein first, so that you know your nutritional needs are met. On the following pages are some tasty go-tos that you will find on many menus.

- Chicken skewers (these are usually on the apps list but make a great dinner)

- Salads: Chicken Caesar (preferably grilled chicken, not breaded) or Cobb

- Omelets and scrambles with a side of fruit

- Burgers (bunless as an option) with all the trimmings—and if it comes with fries, swap in a side salad

- Indian: Tandoori chicken, beef, shrimp, and salmon are great options if you don't have the stomach for heavy or sweet sauces; they're grilled and usually served with mild spices; saag paneer (spinach and Indian cheese)

- Sushi: Sashimi and simple handrolls; miso soup; edamame

- Chinese: Chicken or beef and broccoli; mapo tofu; also most Chinese take-out restaurants have a menu section for steamed meats and vegetable dishes, with sauces available on the side; use rice like a garnish, or steam yourself a bag of riced cauliflower (Trader Joe's and Cascadian Farms are two brands on the market) if you'd rather avoid starchy carbs entirely

- Middle Eastern: Kebabs, salad, eggplant, hummus

- Greek: Salad, yogurt-based dips and sauces such as tzatziki; grilled lamb, fish, and chicken

- Pizza/pasta: Order additional things like Caesar salad or antipasto salad, meatballs, or eggplant rollatini, or you can certainly fork-and-knife the pizza and leave some crust behind. But if it's top-notch stuff and/or you're in Italy, enjoy yourself and return to eating SoWell tomorrow

## Fast-Casual Food

When picking meals to support protein-first eating, take a look at the nutritional info, when available. If the protein value is greater than the carb value, it's a winner.

These days, most chain restaurants and convenience shops cater to customers who want their protein. Some dependable go-tos:

- Chipotle and many other fast-Mexican options allow you to customize your plate, so you can avoid any foods that trigger side effects for you. "Bowl" menu items typically have plenty of protein.

- Starbucks is useful because of its sheer ubiquity, in most US cities and airports. Try the sous vide egg bites, cheese and meat boxes, and egg sandwiches and wraps. Whole-milk lattes offer good nutrition, especially if you add your favorite collagen powder for a protein boost.

- Chick-fil-A has grilled chicken nuggets, a great choice if your stomach won't tolerate breaded nuggets.

- At convenience stores like 7-Eleven, look for hard-boiled eggs, cheese and meat sticks, Greek yogurt, and protein shakes and bars.

## Travel

Travel presents its own challenges, but I've found that with some preparation, it's not difficult to maintain your SoWell eating. My patient Selena frequently has two-week-long business trips that take her to every state in the US. When she finds out where she's staying, she calls and makes sure there's a fridge in her room. If there's not one there already, she tells them she needs one for a medical reason, and she's never had a hotel fail to accommodate the request. On every trip, she packs her blender bottle and protein and a selection of protein bars, meat and cheese sticks, and sometimes even leftovers from the last meal she cooked at home. When she arrives, she goes to the grocery store or places an online order with a local delivery service so that her fridge is stocked with Greek yogurt and her other favorite foods.

With these few prep steps, Selena was able to travel throughout her titration period, and still does so today, without discomfort or much interruption to her usual routine. At restaurants, she chooses an entrée with a protein she likes, and eats the protein first. It's that simple. When possible, she checks out the menu ahead of time and plans her order.

**TRAVEL PREP LIST**

⊕ Call the hotel and request a small refrigerator for your room.

⊕ Pack a "go bag" of your favorite staple snacks.

⊕ Go to the grocery store or place an online order once you arrive.

# In Conclusion

One day while I was writing this book, a patient who had lost 60 pounds thanked me for my help on her journey. It was an emotional moment. She had entered my practice convinced that weight loss was impossible for her; actually, she was really cranky with me on her first visit! But she had come to me anyway, because health problems had convinced her to give it one last try. And now here she was, happily at goal, feeling better than she thought she ever could.

She teared up when she expressed her relief that she would not have to suffer the health consequences of obesity that her mother and grandmother had struggled with in their later years. Then she remembered that I had told her about my own grandmothers' health battles and their role in my decision to enter obesity medicine. "Your grandmothers would be so proud," she said. "I wish that you could have been their doctor and that these medications had been available for them."

I wish that, too. I am so grateful to be part of a new era in medicine that has learned enough about human biology—and about weight stigma—to free us from the idea that *any* kind of weight gain is a personal failure.

GLP-1s are still in their infancy. Even more effective versions of these hormone-based weight-loss drugs are in the pipeline, including an oral version—all of which will have a huge impact on access and, eventually, cost. You are part of a revolution in medicine. We can't change the past, but we hope that we can change the future.

Today, weight prejudice still affects all of us, making the journey to health that much more difficult for so many. I hope each of you sees yourself as a leader, not just in a medical revolution but in a social one. Show the world the SoWell way:

Embrace GLP-1s not as a fad diet, but as a helpful tool to support gentle lifestyle changes that become sustainable healthy habits over time.

Enjoy your body at any size, *and* make evidence-based decisions about weight health.

Practice healthy moderation, without obsession or punitive restriction.

Build a joyful, active lifestyle that fits your body and your preferences.

Celebrate good health as a means to an end—living a long and happy life—in which you can show up strong for the people you care about most.

## I wish you the best on your journey!

Find me online @alexandrasowamd, and join the revolution by becoming part of the SoWell community:

# Appendices

# Food, Lifestyle, and Emotional and Physical Effects Tracker

This log can help you track the events surrounding how and when you eat, and if they connect to your emotions. Make copies, if desired, for multiple days.

For a downloadable or digital version, use this QR code:

# Hunger Scale + Food Log

DATE: _____  ☐ SUN ☐ MON ☐ TUE ☐ WED ☐ THU ☐ FRI ☐ SAT

| TIME | HUNGER (1-10*) | WHAT I ATE AND/OR DRANK | FULLNESS (1-10*) | NOTES (EVENTS AND/OR FEELINGS) |
|------|------|------|------|------|
|  |  |  |  |  |
|  |  |  |  |  |
|  |  |  |  |  |
|  |  |  |  |  |
|  |  |  |  |  |
|  |  |  |  |  |
|  |  |  |  |  |
|  |  |  |  |  |
|  |  |  |  |  |
|  |  |  |  |  |
|  |  |  |  |  |
|  |  |  |  |  |

*Hunger/Fullness Scale | Ideally try to begin eating when your hunger is at a 3-3.5 and stop at 5.

| 1 | 2 | 3 | 4 | 5 | 6 | 7 | 8 | 9 | 10 |
|---|---|---|---|---|---|---|---|---|---|
| Starving, weak, dizzy | Very hungry, low energy, stomach growling a lot | Pretty hungry, stomach is growling a little | Starting to feel a little hungry | Satisfied, neither hungry nor full | A little full, pleasantly full | A little uncomfortable | Feeling stuffed | Very uncomfortable, stomach hurts | So full I feel sick |

# Meal Planner Worksheet

At the start of the day (or night before), plan out your goals for the following categories and make a contingency plan under "24-Hour Plan." At the end of the day, pull out a new sheet and:

1. **"Audit" the day, and**

2. **Create a new plan for tomorrow.**

Try to stay emotionally neutral in creating and evaluating the plan (i.e., don't beat yourself up if not everything goes according to plan).

For a downloadable or digital version, use this QR code:

# Daily Meal Plan & Audit

| BREAKFAST | LUNCH | DINNER |
|---|---|---|
|  |  |  |

| SNACKS | EXERCISE/STRESS MGMT | WATER |
|---|---|---|
|  |  |  |

One word to describe how I feel about my plan:

What I plan to do if my plan gets hard/goes off course:

| What went right today? | What could I have done better? | What will I do better tomorrow? |
|---|---|---|
|  |  |  |

# Cognitive Behavioral Training Tool Kit

For a downloadable
or digital version,
use this QR code:

# Cognitive Behavioral
# Training Tool Kit

**EVENT:** *What happened? What was the thought and what caused it?*

↓

**NEGATIVE THOUGHT/BELIEF:** *What did you tell yourself and what caused it?*

↓

**FEELING:** *How did you feel? What did you feel?*

↓

**ACTION:** *What behavior resulted?*

↓

**CONSEQUENCE:** *What was the result of your action?*

# Rewiring Thoughts:

What can you tell yourself on such occasions in the future? If you have this negative thought again, how can you intentionally rewire your negative thinking?

_____

_____

_____

_____

_____

_____

_____

_____

_____

_____

_____

_____

_____

_____

_____

_____

_____

_____

_____

_____

# Acknowledgments

In the fall of 2023, I had a Zoom meeting with my friend, Territory Foods CEO Ellis McCue, about the evolving and exciting landscape of obesity medicine. I told her about the phenomenal patient outcomes we were having at SoWell Health and she told me, in no uncertain terms, "You need to write a book and share your practice with the world."

The timing couldn't have been worse: I was three months pregnant with my fourth child, had a big product launch in the works, and was running a busy medical practice.

But she was right. That night, I started outlining *The Ozempic Revolution*. Ellis, thank you for always being so generous with your time and talent, and seeing the vision even before I did.

This book would not be possible without two very important groups of people: my patients and my family. To all my patients, but especially to those who shared their stories for the book: Thank you for putting your trust in me and inspiring me every day. You make me a better doctor.

Thank you to my husband and best friend, Peter McPartland, Jr., for encouraging me to always dream bigger, all while creating the most beautiful family together. I could not have picked a better life—and now work—partner. You make me a better person.

To my parents, Dr. David and Karen Sowa, who put no limits on who I could be or what I could achieve. I dreamed of being an author since I was 10 years old; thank you for helping me to grow the knowledge, confidence, and grammar to do so.

I owe a debt of gratitude to all of the people who helped to make this book: My literary agent, Stephanie Tade, for immediately seeing the vision and for being a calming, knowing force during this entire journey; my editor, Deb Brody, for understanding the great need for this book; the entire HarperCollins and Harvest teams, for their support and talent throughout; and finally, my writing collaborator, Sara Grace, who helped me to blend science and softness—I could not have done this without you!

To all of my obesity medicine colleagues, but especially Dr. Louis Aronne, Dr. Melanie Jay, and Dr. Eric Westman, for generously teaching me so much at the very start of my career. A big thank you to Dr. Carolynn Francavilla, for always championing other doctors and for connecting me to Dr. Jesse Richards, whose expert eyes let me breathe a sigh of relief.

And finally, to my SoWell team: Kelly Flanagan, for being my right-hand person over the past three years, and Lo Martin, Lizzie Hays, Caralyn Boivin, Kati Roiz, and Lorena Gonzalez for helping bring SoWell's mission to life. Thank you!

# Notes

## Introduction: Why Doctors Have Failed You

1. Custom Market Insights, *U.S. Weight Loss Market 2024–2033*, April 2023, https://www.custommarketinsights.com/report/us-weight-loss-market/.

2. R. S. Leslie et al., "Real-World Adherence and Persistence to Glucagon-Like Peptide-1 Receptor Agonists among Non-Diabetic Obese Commercially Insured Adults," Prime Therapeutics, https://www.primetherapeutics.com/wp-content/uploads/2024/03/4085-C_AMCP_SP24_GLP-1a-Adherence.pdf.

3. A. Michael Lincoff et al., "Semaglutide and Cardiovascular Outcomes in Obesity without Diabetes," *New England Journal of Medicine* 389, no. 24 (2023): 2221–32; DOI: 10.1056/NEJMoa2307563.

## Chapter 1: Why "Try Harder" Is Terrible Medical Advice

1. Giles S. H. Yeo and Lora K. Heisler, "Unraveling the Brain Regulation of Appetite: Lessons from Genetics," *Nature Neuroscience* 15, no. 10 (2012): 1343–9; DOI: 10.1038/nn.3211.

2. Modified from Gregory J. Morton, Thomas H. Meek, and Michael W. Schwartz, "Neurobiology of Food Intake in Health and Disease," *Nature Reviews Neuroscience* 15, no. 6 (June 2014): 367–78; DOI: 10.1038/nrn3745.

3. Tatiana V. Kirichenko et al., "The Role of Adipokines in Inflammatory Mechanisms of Obesity," *International Journal of Molecular Sciences* 23, no. 23 (November 29, 2022): 14982; DOI: 10.3390/ijms232314982.

4. Milan Obradovic et al., "Leptin and Obesity: Role and Clinical Implication," *Frontiers in Endocrinology* 12 (May 18, 2021): 585887; DOI: 10.3389/fendo.2021.585887.

5. Ilia N. Karatsoreos et al., "Food for Thought: Hormonal, Experiential, and Neural Influences on Feeding and Obesity," *Journal of Neuroscience* 33, no. 45 (November 6, 2013): 17610–6; DOI: 10.1523/JNEUROSCI.3452-13.2013.

6. Priya Sumithran et al., "Long-Term Persistence of Hormonal Adaptations to Weight Loss," *New England Journal of Medicine* 365, no. 17 (2011): 1597–604; DOI: 10.1056/NEJMoa1105816.

7. Luca Busetto et al., "Mechanisms of Weight Regain," *European Journal of Internal Medicine* 93 (2021): 3–7; DOI: 10.1016/j.ejim.2021.01.002.

8. Erin Fothergill et al., "Persistent Metabolic Adaptation 6 Years After 'The Biggest Loser' Competition," *Obesity* (Silver Spring, MD) 24, no. 8 (2016): 1612–9; DOI: 10.1002/oby.21538.

9. Albert J. Stunkard et al., "The Body-Mass Index of Twins Who Have Been Reared Apart," *New England Journal of Medicine* 322, no. 21 (1990): 1483–7; DOI: 10.1056/NEJM199005243222102.

10. Albert J. Stunkard et al., "An Adoption Study of Human Obesity," *New England Journal of Medicine* 314, no. 4 (1986): 193–8; DOI: 10.1056/NEJM198601233140401.

11. Jessica Duis and Merlin G. Butler, "Syndromic and Nonsyndromic Obesity: Underlying Genetic Causes in Humans," *Advanced Biology* 6, no. 10 (October 2022): e2101154; DOI: 10.1002/adbi.202101154.

12. C. M. Hales et al., "Prevalence of Obesity and Severe Obesity Among Adults: United States, 2017–2018," NCHS Data Brief, no 360 (Hyattsville, MD: National Center for Health Statistics), 2020; Cynthia L. Ogden and Margaret D. Carroll, "Prevalence of Overweight, Obesity, and Extreme Obesity Among Adults: United States, Trends 1960–1962 Through 2007–2008," Division of Health and Nutrition Examination Surveys.

13. Elizabeth Blackburn, *The Telomere Effect: A Revolutionary Approach to Living Younger, Healthier, Longer* (New York: Hachette, 2017), 6.

14. C. D. Fryar et al., "Prevalence of Overweight, Obesity, and Severe Obesity Among Adults Aged 20 and Over: United States, 1960–1962 Through 2017–2018," NCHS Health E-Stats, 2020.

15. John G. Kral et al., "Large Maternal Weight Loss from Obesity Surgery Prevents Transmission of Obesity to Children Who Were Followed for 2 to 18 Years," *Pediatrics* 118, no. 6 (2006): e1644–9; DOI: 10.1542/peds.2006-1379.

16. Zachary J. Ward et al., "Projected U.S. State-Level Prevalence of Adult Obesity and Severe Obesity," *New England Journal of Medicine* 381, no. 25 (2019): 2440–50; DOI: 10.1056/NEJMsa1909301.

## Chapter 2: How GLP-1s Reverse Obesity, End Yo-Yo Dieting, and Protect You from Disease

1. Joana Araújo et al., "Prevalence of Optimal Metabolic Health in American Adults: National Health and Nutrition Examination Survey 2009–2016," *Metabolic Syndrome and Related Disorders* 17, no. 1 (2019): 46–52; DOI: 10.1089/met.2018.0105.

2. Julio Rosenstock et al., "Efficacy and Safety of a Novel Dual GIP and GLP-1 Receptor Agonist Tirzepatide in Patients with Type 2 Diabetes (SURPASS-1): A Double-Blind, Randomised, Phase 3 Trial," *Lancet* (London, England) 398, no. 10295 (2021): 143–55; DOI: 10.1016/S0140-6736(21)01324-6.

3. Anita Slomski, "Obesity Is Now the Top Modifiable Dementia Risk Factor in the US," *JAMA* 328, no. 1 (2022): 10; DOI: 10.1001/jama.2022.11058.

4. William Wang et al., "Associations of Semaglutide with Incidence and Recurrence of Alcohol Use Disorder in Real-World Population," *Nature Communications* 15, no. 1 (May 28, 2024): 4548; DOI: 10.1038/s41467-024-48780-6.

5. Jeanna Vazquez, "Clinical Trial Studying Possible New Treatment Option for Patients with NAFLD," UC San Diego Health, August 23, 2023, https://health.ucsd.edu/news/press-releases/2023-08-23-clinical-trial-studying-possible-new-treatment-option-for-patients-with-nafld/.

6. Vlado Perkovic et al., "Effects of Semaglutide on Chronic Kidney Disease in Patients with Type 2 Diabetes," *New England Journal of Medicine* 391, no. 2 (July 11, 2024): 109–21; DOI: 10.1056/NEJMoa2403347.

7. Atul Malhotra et al., "Tirzepatide for the Treatment of Obstructive Sleep Apnea: Rationale, Design, and Sample Baseline Characteristics of the SURMOUNT-OSA Phase 3 Trial," *Contemporary Clinical Trials* 141 (June 2024): 107516; DOI: 10.1016/j.cct.2024.107516.

8. C. H. Nørgaard et al., "Treatment with Glucagon-Like Peptide-1 Receptor Agonists and Incidence of Dementia: Data from Pooled Double-Blind Randomized Controlled Trials and Nationwide Disease and Prescription Registers," *Alzheimer's & Dementia* 8, no. 1 (2022): e12268; DOI: 10.1002/trc2.12268.

## Chapter 3: What the GLP-1 Experience Really Feels Like: An FAQ

1. Ania M. Jastreboff et al., "Tirzepatide Once Weekly for the Treatment of Obesity," *New England Journal of Medicine* 387, no. 3 (July 21, 2022): 205–16, DOI: 10.1056/NEJMoa2206038; John P. H. Wilding et al., "Once-Weekly Semaglutide in Adults with Overweight or Obesity," *New England Journal of Medicine* 384, no. 11 (March 18, 2021): 989–1002; DOI: 10.1056/NEJMoa2032183.

2. Melanie J. Davies et al., "Efficacy of Liraglutide for Weight Loss Among Patients with Type 2 Diabetes: The SCALE Diabetes Randomized Clinical Trial," *JAMA* 314, no. 7 (August 18, 2015): 687–99; DOI: 10.1001/jama.2015.9676.

3. Jastreboff et al., "Tirzepatide Once Weekly for the Treatment of Obesity."

4. W. Timothy Garvey et al., "Tirzepatide Once Weekly for the Treatment of Obesity in People with Type 2 Diabetes (SURMOUNT-2): A Double-Blind, Randomised, Multicentre, Placebo-Controlled, Phase 3 Trial," *Lancet* 402, no. 10402 (August 19, 2023): 613–26; DOI: 0.1016/S0140-6736(23)01200-X.

5. Wilding et al., "Once-Weekly Semaglutide in Adults with Overweight or Obesity."

6. Melanie Davies et al., "Semaglutide 2.4 mg Once a Week in Adults with Overweight or Obesity, and Type 2 Diabetes (STEP 2): A Randomised, Double-Blind, Double Dummy, Placebo-Controlled, Phase 3 Trial," *Lancet* 397, no. 10278 (March 13, 2021): 971-84; DOI: 10.1016/S0140-6736(21)00213-0.

7. Mojca Jensterle et al., "Efficacy of GLP-1 RA Approved for Weight Management in Patients With or Without Diabetes: A Narrative Review," *Advances in Therapy* 39, no. 6 (2022): 2452–67; DOI: 10.1007/s12325-022-02153-x.

8. Orlistat: Jarl S. Torgerson et al., "XENical in the Prevention of Diabetes in Obese Subjects (XENDOS) Study: A Randomized Study of Orlistat as an Adjunct to Lifestyle Changes for the Prevention of Type 2 Diabetes in Obese Patients," *Diabetes Care* 27, no. 1 (2004): 155–61; DOI: 10.2337/diacare.27.1.155.

9. Metformin: R. A. DeFronzo and A. M. Goodman, "Efficacy of Metformin in Patients with Non-Insulin-Dependent Diabetes Mellitus. The Multicenter Metformin Study Group," *New England Journal of Medicine* 333, no. 9 (1995): 541–9; DOI: 10.1056/NEJM199508313330902.

10. Naltrexone/Bupropion and Phentermine/Topirimate: Rohan Khera et al., "Association of Pharmacological Treatments for Obesity with Weight Loss and Adverse Events: A Systematic Review and Meta-Analysis," *JAMA* 315, no. 22 (2016): 2424–34; DOI: 10.1001/jama.2016.7602.

11. Liraglutide: Julie R. Lundgren et al., "Healthy Weight Loss Maintenance with Exercise, Liraglutide, or Both Combined," *New England Journal of Medicine* 384, no. 18 (2021): 1719–1730; DOI: 10.1056/NEJMoa2028198.

12. Semaglutide: John P. H. Wilding et al., "Once-Weekly Semaglutide in Adults with Overweight or Obesity," *New England Journal of Medicine* 384, no. 11 (2021): 989–1002; DOI: 10.1056/NEJMoa2032183.

13. Ania M. Jastreboff et al., "Tirzepatide Once Weekly for the Treatment of Obesity."

14. Jensterle et al., "Efficacy of GLP-1 RA Approved for Weight Management in Patients With or Without Diabetes: A Narrative Review."

15. Louis J. Aronne et al., "Continued Treatment with Tirzepatide for Maintenance of Weight Reduction in Adults with Obesity: The SURMOUNT-4 Randomized Clinical Trial," *JAMA* 331, no. 1 (2024): 38–48; DOI: 10.1001/jama.2023.24945.

16. Davies et al., "Semaglutide 2.4 mg Once a Week in Adults with Overweight or Obesity, and Type 2 Diabetes (STEP 2)."

17. Sean Wharton et al., "Managing the Gastrointestinal Side Effects of GLP-1 Receptor Agonists in Obesity: Recommendations for Clinical Practice," *Postgraduate Medicine* 134, no. 1 (2022): 14–9; DOI: 10.1080/00325481.2021.2002616.

18. Sean Wharton et al., "Two-Year Effect of Semaglutide 2.4 mg on Control of Eating in Adults with Overweight/Obesity: STEP 5," *Obesity* (Silver Spring, MD) 31, no. 3 (2023): 703–15; DOI: 10.1002/oby.23673.

19. W. Timothy Garvey et al., "Two-Year Effects of Semaglutide in Adults with Overweight or Obesity: The STEP 5 Trial," *Nature Medicine* 28, no. 10 (2022): 2083–91; DOI: 10.1038/s41591-022-02026-4; Donna H. Ryan et al., "Long-Term Weight Loss Effects of Semaglutide in Obesity Without Diabetes in the SELECT Trial," *Nature Medicine* 30 (May 13, 2024): 2049–57; DOI: 10.1038/s41591-024-02996-7.

20. John P H Wilding et al. "Weight regain and cardiometabolic effects after withdrawal of semaglutide: The STEP 1 trial extension." *Diabetes, Obesity & Metabolism* vol. 24,8 (2022): 1553-1564. DOI: 10.1111/dom.14725.

21. Domenica Rubino et al., "Effect of Continued Weekly Subcutaneous Semaglutide vs Placebo on Weight Loss Maintenance in Adults with Overweight or Obesity: The STEP 4 Randomized Clinical Trial," *JAMA* 325, no. 14 (2021): 1414–25; DOI: 10.1001/jama.2021.32220.

22. Akua Nuako et al., "Pharmacologic Treatment of Obesity in Reproductive Aged Women," *Current Obstetrics and Gynecology Reports* 12, no. 2 (2023): 138–46; DOI: 10.1007/s13669-023-00350-1.

23. Amy Klein, "An Ozempic Baby Boom? Some GLP-1 Users Report Unexpected Pregnancies," *Washington Post*, April 5, 2024, https://www.washingtonpost.com/wellness/2024/04/05/ozempic-babies-weight-loss-fertility/.

24. R. L. Weinsier et al., "Medically Safe Rate of Weight Loss for the Treatment of Obesity: A Guideline Based on Risk of Gallstone Formation," *American Journal of Medicine* 98, no. 2 (1995): 115–7; DOI: 10.1016/S0002-9343(99)80394-5.

25. Sang-Yong Son et al., "Prevention of Gallstones After Bariatric Surgery Using Ursodeoxycholic Acid: A Narrative Review of Literatures," *Journal of Metabolic and Bariatric Surgery* 11, no. 2 (2022): 30-8; DOI: 10.17476/jmbs.2022.11.2.30.

26. Vicky Ka Ming Li et al., "Predictors of Gallstone Formation After Bariatric Surgery: A Multivariate Analysis of Risk Factors Comparing Gastric Bypass, Gastric Banding, and Sleeve Gastrectomy," *Surgical Endoscopy* 23, no. 7 (2009): 1640–4; DOI: 10.1007/s00464-008-0204-6.

27. Liyun He et al., "Association of Glucagon-Like Peptide-1 Receptor Agonist Use with Risk of Gallbladder and Biliary Diseases: A Systematic Review and Meta-analysis of Randomized Clinical Trials," *JAMA Internal Medicine* 182, no. 5 (2022): 513–9; DOI: 10.1001/jamainternmed.2022.0338.

28. Chuqing Cao et al., "GLP-1 Receptor Agonists and Pancreatic Safety Concerns in Type 2 Diabetic Patients: Data from Cardiovascular Outcome Trials," *Endocrine* 68, no. 3 (2020): 518–25; DOI: 10.1007/s12020-020-02223-6.

29. Rachel Dankner et al., "Glucagon-Like Peptide-1 Receptor Agonists and Pancreatic Cancer Risk in Patients with Type 2 Diabetes," *JAMA Network Open* 7, no. 1 (January 2, 2024): e2350408; DOI: 10.1001/jamanetworkopen.2023.50408.

30. Garvey et al., "Two-Year Effects of Semaglutide in Adults with Overweight or Obesity: The STEP 5 Trial."

31. Aronne et al., "Continued Treatment with Tirzepatide for Maintenance of Weight Reduction in Adults with Obesity: The SURMOUNT-4 Randomized Clinical Trial."

32. Mohit Sodhi et al., "Risk of Gastrointestinal Adverse Events Associated with Glucagon-Like Peptide-1 Receptor Agonists for Weight Loss," *JAMA* 330, no. 18 (2023): 1795–7; DOI: 10.1001/jama.2023.19574.

33. William Wang et al., "Association of Semaglutide with Risk of Suicidal Ideation in a Real-World Cohort," *Nature Medicine* 30, 1 (2024): 168–76; DOI: 10.1038/s41591-023-02672-2.

## Chapter 4: Are You a Candidate for a GLP-1?

1. Chi Pang Wen et al., "Are Asians at Greater Mortality Risks for Being Overweight Than Caucasians? Redefining Obesity for Asians," *Public Health Nutrition* 12, no. 4 (2009): 497–506; DOI: 10.1017/S1368980008002802.

## Chapter 5: The Habit Foundations

1. Adapted from *You Count, Calories Don't*, by Linda Omichinski with Mary Evans Young (London: Hodder & Stoughton, 1992).

## Chapter 6: The Food Foundations

1. Matt Reynolds, "What the Scientists Who Pioneered Weight-Loss Drugs Want You to Know," *Wired*, June 12, 2023, https://www.wired.com/story/obesity-drugs-researcher-interview-ozempic-wegovy/. Accessed June 18, 2024.

2. Alpana P. Shukla et al., "Food Order Has a Significant Impact on Postprandial Glucose and Insulin Levels," *Diabetes Care* 38, no. 7 (2015): e98–9; DOI: 10.2337/dc15-0429.

3. John W. Carbone et al., "Recent Advances in the Characterization of Skeletal Muscle and Whole-Body Protein Responses to Dietary Protein and Exercise During Negative Energy Balance," *Advances in Nutrition* (Bethesda, MD) 10, no. 1 (2019): 70–9; DOI: 10.1093/advances/nmy087.

4. Anita Belza et al., "Contribution of Gastroenteropancreatic Appetite Hormones to Protein-Induced Satiety," *American Journal of Clinical Nutrition* 97, no. 5 (2013): 980–9; DOI: 10.3945/ajcn.112.047563.

5. Jaecheol Moon and Gwanpyo Koh, "Clinical Evidence and Mechanisms of High-Protein Diet-Induced Weight Loss," *Journal of Obesity & Metabolic Syndrome* 29, no. 3 (2020): 166–73; DOI: 10.7570/jomes20028.

6. Sebely Pal and Vanessa Ellis, "The Acute Effects of Four Protein Meals on Insulin, Glucose, Appetite and Energy Intake in Lean Men," *British Journal of Nutrition* 104, no. 8 (2010): 1241–8; DOI: 10.1017/S0007114510001911.

7. Stuart M. Phillips et al., "The Role of Milk- and Soy-Based Protein in Support of Muscle Protein Synthesis and Muscle Protein Accretion in Young and Elderly Persons," *Journal of the American College of Nutrition* 28, no. 4 (2009): 343–54; DOI: 10.1080/07315724.2009.10718096.

8. E. Proksch et al., "Oral Supplementation of Specific Collagen Peptides Has Beneficial Effects on Human Skin Physiology: A Double-Blind, Placebo-Controlled Study," *Skin Pharmacology and Physiology* 27, no. 1 (2014): 47–55; DOI: 10.1159/000351376; Patrick Jendricke et al., "Specific Collagen Peptides in Combination with Resistance Training Improve Body Composition and Regional Muscle Strength in Premenopausal Women: A Randomized Controlled Trial," *Nutrients* 11, no. 4 (April 20, 2019): 892; DOI: 10.3390/nu11040892.

## Chapter 7: The Mental Foundations

1. Wiremu Hohaia et al., "Occipital Alpha-Band Brain Waves When the Eyes Are Closed Are Shaped by Ongoing Visual Processes," *Scientific Reports* 12, no. 1 (January 24, 2022): 1194; DOI: 10.1038/s41598-022-05289-6.

Chapter 9: Getting a Prescription and Getting It Covered

1. U.S. Food and Drug Administration, "Compounded Drug Products That Are Essentially Copies of a Commercially Available Drug Product Under Section 503A of the Federal Food, Drug, and Cosmetic Act—Guidance for Industry," January 2018, https://www.fda.gov/files/drugs/published/Compounded-Drug-Products-That-Are-Essentially-Copies-of-a-Commercially-Available-Drug-Product-Under-Section-503A-of-the-Federal-Food--Drug--and-Cosmetic-Act-Guidance-for-Industry.pdf.

Chapter 10: Why Hard Cardio Can Hurt—and What to Do Instead

1. Carla E. Cox, "Role of Physical Activity for Weight Loss and Weight Maintenance," *Diabetes Spectrum* 30, no. 3 (August 2017): 157–60; DOI: 10.2337/ds17-0013.

2. James A. Levine, "Nonexercise Activity Thermogenesis (NEAT): Environment and Biology," *American Journal of Physiology, Endocrinology and Metabolism* 286, no. 5 (2004): E675–85; DOI: 10.1152/ajpendo.00562.2003.

3. Christian von Loeffelholz and Andreas L. Birkenfeld, "Non-Exercise Activity Thermogenesis in Human Energy Homeostasis," in *Endotext*, ed. Kenneth R. Feingold et al. (MDText.com, Inc., 2022).

4. Bokun Kim et al., "Changes in Muscle Strength After Diet-Induced Weight Reduction in Adult Men with Obesity: A Prospective Study," *Diabetes, Metabolic Syndrome and Obesity: Targets and Therapy* 10 (May 9, 2017): 187–94; DOI: 10.2147/DMSO.S132707.

5. Zimian Wang et al., "Specific Metabolic Rates of Major Organs and Tissues Across Adulthood: Evaluation by Mechanistic Model of Resting Energy Expenditure," *American Journal of Clinical Nutrition* 92, no. 6 (2010): 1369–77; DOI: 10.3945/ajcn.2010.29885.

6. Xiaoming Zhang et al., "Association of Sarcopenic Obesity with the Risk of All-Cause Mortality Among Adults Over a Broad Range of Different Settings: A Updated Meta-Analysis," *BMC Geriatrics* 19, no. 1 (July 3, 2019): 183; DOI: 10.1186/s12877-019-1195-y.

7. Gretchen Reynolds, "The Scientific 7-Minute Workout," *New York Times*, May 9, 2013, https://nyti.ms/3s5swHj. Accessed June 21, 2024.

8. Robert W. Morton et al., "Neither Load nor Systemic Hormones Determine Resistance Training-Mediated Hypertrophy or Strength Gains in Resistance-Trained Young Men," *Journal of Applied Physiology* (Bethesda, MD) 121, no. 1 (2016): 129–38; DOI: 10.1152/japplphysiol.00154.2016.

9. Thomas M. Longland et al., "Higher Compared with Lower Dietary Protein During an Energy Deficit Combined with Intense Exercise Promotes Greater Lean Mass Gain and Fat Mass Loss: A Randomized Trial," *American Journal of Clinical Nutrition* 103, no. 3 (2016): 738–46; DOI: 10.3945/ajcn.115.119339.

10. Berit Østergaard Christoffersen et al., "Beyond Appetite Regulation: Targeting Energy Expenditure, Fat Oxidation, and Lean Mass Preservation for Sustainable Weight Loss," *Obesity* (Silver Spring, MD) 30, no. 4 (2022): 841–857; DOI: 10.1002/oby.23374.

11. John Blundell et al., "Effects of Once-Weekly Semaglutide on Appetite, Energy Intake, Control of Eating, Food Preference and Body Weight in Subjects with Obesity," *Diabetes, Obesity & Metabolism* 19, no. 9 (2017): 1242–51; DOI: 10.1111/dom.12932; Ania M. Jastreboff et al., "Tirzepatide Once Weekly for the Treatment of Obesity," *New England Journal of Medicine* 387, no. 3 (2022): 205–16; DOI: 10.1056/NEJMoa2206038.

12. M. L. Klem et al., "A Descriptive Study of Individuals Successful at Long-Term Maintenance of Substantial Weight Loss," *American Journal of Clinical Nutrition* 66, no. 2 (1997): 239–46; DOI: 10.1093/ajcn/66.2.239.

13. Marie H. Murphy et al., "The Effects of Continuous Compared to Accumulated Exercise on Health: A Meta-Analytic Review," *Sports Medicine* (Auckland, NZ) 49, no. 10 (2019): 1585–607; DOI: 10.1007/s40279-019-01145-2.

14. Tobias Engeroff et al., "After Dinner Rest a While, After Supper Walk a Mile? A Systematic Review with Meta-analysis on the Acute Postprandial Glycemic Response to Exercise Before and After Meal Ingestion in Healthy Subjects and Patients with Impaired Glucose Tolerance," *Sports Medicine* (Auckland, NZ) 53, no. 4 (2023): 849–69; DOI: 10.1007/s40279-022-01808-7.

15. Karlijn Burridge et al., "Obesity History, Physical Exam, Laboratory, Body Composition, and Energy Expenditure: An Obesity Medicine Association (OMA) Clinical Practice Statement (CPS) 2022," *Obesity Pillars* 1 (January 10, 2022): 100007; DOI: 10.1016/j.obpill.2021.100007.

16. Clifton J. Holmes and Susan B. Racette, "The Utility of Body Composition Assessment in Nutrition and Clinical Practice: An Overview of Current Methodology," *Nutrients* 13, no. 8 (July 22, 2021): 2493; DOI: 10.3390/nu13082493.

17. Madelin R. Siedler et al., "Assessing the Reliability and Cross-Sectional and Longitudinal Validity of Fifteen Bioelectrical Impedance Analysis Devices," *British Journal of Nutrition* 130, no. 5 (2023): 827–40; DOI: 10.1017/S0007114522003749.

Chapter 11: Maintaining for Life

1. Girish P. Joshi et al., "American Society of Anesthesiologists Consensus-Based Guidance on Preoperative Management of Patients (Adults and Children) on Glucagon-like Peptide-1 (GLP-1) Receptor Agonists," American Society of Anesthesiologists, June 29, 2023, https://www.asahq.org/about-asa/newsroom/news-releases/2023/06/american-society-of-anesthesiologists-consensus-based-guidance-on-Preoperative.

# Index

# About the Author

Alexandra Sowa, MD, is a trailblazer in obesity medicine, known for her unique blend of scientific rigor and thoughtful patient advocacy. Her dual certification in internal medicine and obesity medicine, along with her education at Johns Hopkins, NYU, and Yale, sets her apart as an expert deeply committed to advancing treatment paradigms. Through SoWell Health, she extends her reach beyond the clinic, offering innovative telehealth services, products, and resources that reflect her philosophy of care—holistic, evidence-based, and deeply respectful of the emotional dimensions of health. She lives in Summit, New Jersey, with her husband and four young children.